Dr. You

Discovering Health and Meaning
Through Empowered Self-Care

DAVID W. BALL, MD

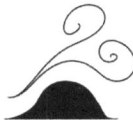

Windy Hill
Publishing

Tyler, Tx

DR. YOU

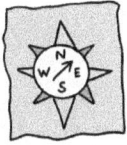

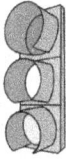

(Awareness)

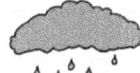
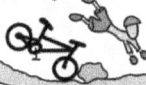

(Adversity)

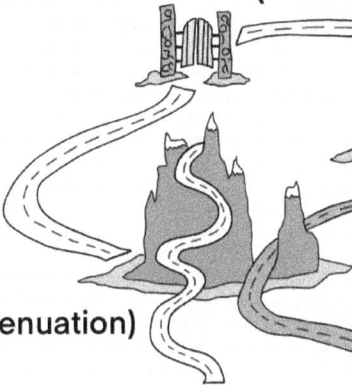

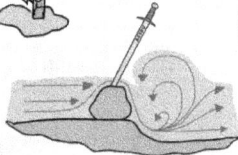

(Attenuation)

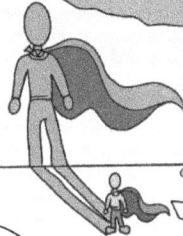

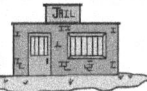

(Assets)

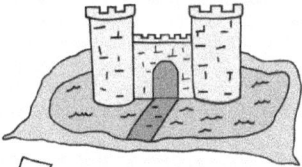

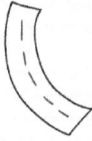

(Allies)

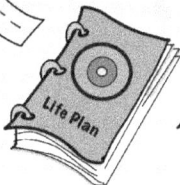

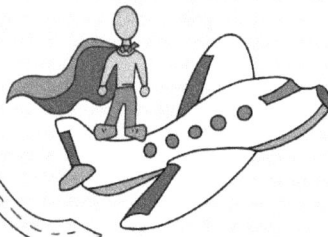

(Aim)

(Action)

Published in the United States of America

ISBN hardcover: 979-8-9870507-1-2
ISBN paperback: 979-8-9870507-0-5

Published by Windy Hill Publishing
Tyler, Texas

www.DrYou.org

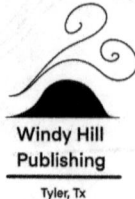

**Windy Hill
Publishing**
Tyler, Tx

Acknowledgments

*To Sara, my wife, for tolerating my incessant conversations
and for walking through life beside me.*

*To my children, Taylor, Spencer and Haley, for
inspiring me to be a better version of myself.*

To Mike Jones for all the inspiring books, support and friendship.

*To my Mother and Father for teaching me the
importance of lifelong learning.*

*To Jeff Goins for believing in the project and building
an editorial team to help me complete the book.*

*To all those who contributed to raising the younger
version of myself—you know who you are.*

Table of Contents

How to Read This Book

Reading, writing and health are similar.
The more intentional you are, the better the outcome.

The key to reading any book is to appropriately match your time and effort to the complexity of the material. Not all books are created equal, so some require more effort than others to consume and understand. The latest fictional spy novel read for entertainment needs only a superficial level of reading. To read and understand Albert Einstein's *On the Method of Theoretical Physics* requires a much more deliberate analytical approach. Only you can decide how much time and effort is appropriate to invest in a book.

If you are not familiar with the basic concepts introduced in this book, you may feel a little overwhelmed. If this is you or if you are simply trying to decide how much time and effort to invest in this book, you may consider a method I learned from Mortimer J. Adler in his book, *How to Read a Book: The Classic Guide to Intelligent Reading.* Interestingly, Adler notes a significant similarity in reading, writing and health. The more intentional you are, the better the outcome.

"Some books are to be tasted, others to be swallowed, and some few to be chewed and digested."[1]

First Stage: Superficial Reading

The goal of superficial reading is to determine whether the book merits a more in-depth read.

a. Reread the title and subtitle.

b. Read the preface.

c. Study the table of contents. Think of this as a map to the journey the book promises.

d. Read the publisher's comments, if any are given.

e. Select the chapters that seem important and quickly inspect them, especially the summary statements at the beginning or end.

f. Briefly thumb through the other chapters and sample various paragraphs and pages. Don't forget to read the last few pages of the book. Authors typically summarize the most important points there.

When you finish this first stage, you should have a good grasp of the book's central ideas and how much time and effort you want to invest. If this is as deep as you think the book merits, stop here. If you are intrigued and want to dive deeper, proceed to the second stage.

Second Stage: Active Reading

The goal of this stage is not just to accumulate information, but to gain a thorough understanding. As such, it is more effortful than the first stage.

---

1   Francis Bacon, *Complete Essays* (Dover Publications, 2008).

a. Classify the book. Based on your superficial reading, categorize the book into an appropriate genre.

b. Briefly summarize the book in a couple of sentences.

c. Outline the major parts.

d. State the problem(s) the author is attempting to solve.

e. Understand the author's terms, words and phrases in their appropriate context.

f. Identify the core arguments.

g. Summarize the author's solutions.

h. Remain curious and avoid passing judgment until you understand what the author is trying to communicate.

i. Make your critique. Intellectual criticism is not based on opinion alone. You must provide reasons for your critique. If you feel the author's arguments are incorrect, explain how the book is:

    1. Uninformed

    2. Misinformed

    3. Illogical

    4. Incomplete

As with most things, your questions are more important than the information in the book. Four big questions to ask are:

- What is the book about?

- What are the details?

- Is it true?

- What now?

If you find the author's message compelling and true, then you must ask, "What will I do about it?" or, "What now?" Knowing information without acting is of little value. As Adler said, "Nothing short of the doing solves the problem."[2] Psychologists are often known to say that you can't think yourself to health; you must do something.

Practical Tips for Active Reading

If you have decided that this book warrants a more in-depth active read, consider these tips to help you grasp and consume the information.

1. Highlight, underline and/or circle the key passages, phrases and words that you find most helpful and interesting.

2. Make notes in the margins. Your own spontaneous questions, thoughts and ideas that arise as you process any book are the most important things any good author can help you discover. I have designed this book intentionally with extra room in the margins so you have ample space to capture these. The blank spaces and pages at the end of the chapters are also good places to capture your thoughts.

3. Dog-ear or mark pages with Post-it Note tabs. This helps you quickly identify passages you feel are most worthy of review.

4. Connect ideas from different sections of the book by noting page numbers in the margins.

5. Connect the ideas from different passages of other books in the margins.

6. Mark important ideas with stars, asterisks, dots or checkmarks.

7. Number key sequential concepts and topics to help highlight their order.

---

2   Mortimer Adler and Charles Van Doren, *How to Read A Book: The Classic Guide to Intelligent Reading* (Touchstone, 1940).

When I finish a good book, the pages are wrinkled and stained with ink. My favorite books are so tattered that if I recommend them to someone, they always want a fresh copy for themselves because my notes, dog-ears and highlights are too distracting.

Once I finish a good book, I review all my notes and highlights. I then take it one step further and record the most important ideas in the GoodNotes app on my iPad. This allows me to study them anywhere and anytime.

Repetitively analyzing and savoring information is one way to communicate to your brain that this information is important and should be stored for long-term use. Information integrated into your brain's long-term memory has the greatest impact on your decisions, behaviors, attitudes, and feelings.

Empowered Self-Care Partners

Another tip to help convert a book's most important concepts into concrete action is to invite someone else to read and work through the book with you. As with any adventure, the journey of building a better life is more enjoyable and rewarding if you share it with another person. Creating shared memories is always more powerful than indulging in solitary ones.

If you choose to start a small group, consider limiting it to ten people or fewer. Studies suggest that once groups get much larger than that, people stop sharing their intimate thoughts and feelings.

These small groups will not only make the reading process more memorable and fun, but the members can also act as accountability partners and sources of encouragement. Partners also help us feel safe when we reach obstacles that make us vulnerable. After all, most people falter in moments of discomfort. Use these times as beacons to guide your path. Think of vulnerability as marking the way to success. We will discuss the details of how to establish and organize these types of small groups in Chapter 6: Allies.

Introduction

Most people think: knowledge solves problems.

The truth is: consistent application of knowledge solves problems.

"I don't really understand myself, for I want to do what is right, but I don't do it. Instead, I do what I hate."[3]

"Knowledge is only potential power. It becomes power only when, and if it is organized into definite plans of action, and directed to a definite end."[4]

C arrie has been healthy her entire life. The only time she goes to her primary care physician is once a year when she gets a sinus infection. Her doctor spends about five minutes with her, just long enough to diagnose her and write an antibiotic prescription. This time is different. Carrie has felt fatigued and unusually thirsty for several weeks, but doesn't know why. She expects her doctor to spend a little more time with her, but as usual he's in and out before she can ask any questions. As he walks out the door, he tells her he is going to run a few tests.

---

3 New Living Translation, Romans 7:15.

4 Napoleon Hill, *Think and Grow Rich* (Simon and Brown, 2010).

A couple of days later, a nurse calls Carrie and tells her she has diabetes. Carrie is shocked. Nobody in her family has diabetes. She has a friend who gives herself insulin shots, but that's the extent of Carrie's knowledge of the condition. The nurse is kind, but only gives her simple instructions. She says that her doctor called in a medication she should take twice a day and she should exercise regularly, eat fewer simple carbohydrates and lose weight.

Three months later, Carrie goes back to see her doctor and discovers that her glucose has worsened. Instead of losing weight, she gained four pounds. Her doctor increases her medication and reiterates that she needs to exercise more, eat fewer carbs and lose weight. He refers her to a diabetic educator who helps her understand what diabetes is, why people develop it, how to treat it, and potential complications if it is not controlled. Loaded with good information, Carrie sets out with new fervor. At first she loses a few pounds and her glucose improves, but after a few months she falls back into her usual routine.

A couple of years after the initial diagnosis, Carrie's diabetes is still not controlled, despite three different medications and hours of "education." Carrie becomes frustrated and stops trying. She laments, "I know what I need to do, but I just can't seem to do it." Ever feel that way?

The Pareto Principle

Carrie's story plays out thousands of times across the United States every day. Our healthcare system wastes trillions of dollars throwing supplements, medications and information at chronic health problems with little effect. Why?

The central thrust of the problem was first described in the early 1900s by Vilfredo Pareto. Legend has it that Pareto—an Italian economist, physicist, mathematician, and philosopher—observed that 20 percent of the pea plants in his garden generated 80 percent of the healthy pods. He noted that this simple ratio repeated itself in a spectrum of human institutions, such as with the distribution of Italy's wealth. Eighty percent of Italy's land was owned by 20 percent of the population. In every society ever studied, regardless of the form of government, this same distribution of wealth is noted. In modern manufacturing, 80 percent of production comes from 20 percent of companies. In language, about 90 percent of communication uses just 500 words. Twenty percent of salespeople generate 80 percent of sales. In retail 20 percent of customers account for 80 percent of total profits. Some call this the 80/20 principle, but it is not about an exact percentage. Sometimes in the real world, the actual percentages look more like 90/10, 75/25 or even 60/40.

The Pareto Principle incorporates two ideas:

- First, the 80 percent. This represents the **Big Problem** that drives the ultimate outcome. It is either solved by or caused by a minority of Key Factors.

- Second, the 20 percent. This minority represents the **Key Factors** that disproportionately contribute to the Big Problem. Master these first and you can change the overall outcome more quickly and effectively.

The Pareto Principle can be found in many instances in our medical system. For example, in developed countries worldwide, 75 percent of premature deaths are caused by chronic disease—**The Big Problem.** Only a handful of diseases—**The Key Factors**—lead to premature death: coronary artery disease, diabetes, chronic lung disease, strokes, cancers, chronic kidney disease, and Alzheimer's disease. We also see the Pareto Principle in how we spend our healthcare dollars. According to the Center for Disease Control, in the United States 75

Premature Death

Acute
Disease

Chronic
Disease

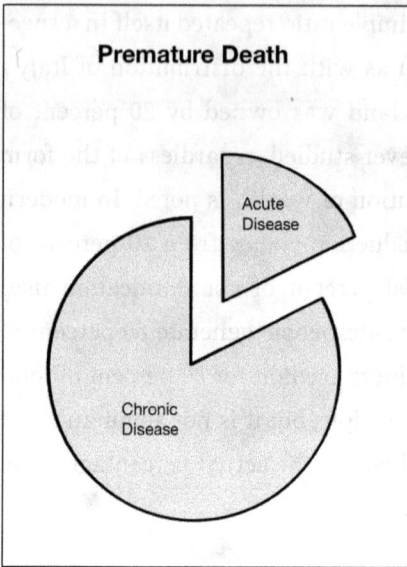

percent of our healthcare budget is spent on these chronic diseases.[5]

Even in developing countries, where communicable diseases are much more prevalent, 70 percent of deaths are now caused by chronic diseases.[6]

If such a large portion of premature deaths are from chronic diseases and across the world our healthcare budgets are exploding, maybe we need to pay more attention to the 20 percent of diseases that cause 80 percent of the premature deaths.

Just as the Pareto Principle predicted that a small number of diseases cause the majority of premature deaths, it can help us focus on a small number of key factors that cause these diseases.

In general, three broad classes of factors cause the majority of chronic diseases: environmental pathogens, genetic factors and unhealthy behaviors. Of the three, one is **The Big Problem,** causing the majority of disease. Can you guess which one?

By a large majority, unhealthy behaviors lead the pack. Of all the unhealthy behaviors that mankind pursues, four cause the majority of illness: smoking, inactivity, poor nutrition, and excessive alcohol consumption. These are the **Key Factors.**

---

5   The Power of Prevention: Chronic Disease the Public Challenge of the 21st Century (Centers For Disease Control and Prevention, 2009).

6   Drue H. Barrett, et al., *Public Health Ethics: Cases Spanning the Globe* (Springer, 1st ed. 2016 edition).

So if we know the four key behaviors that result in the majority of premature deaths worldwide, why are we losing the battle?

The problem boils down to Carrie's last statement and how our healthcare systems address it. Remember what Carrie told us, "I know what I need to do, but I just can't seem to do it."

The problem and the answer is choice.

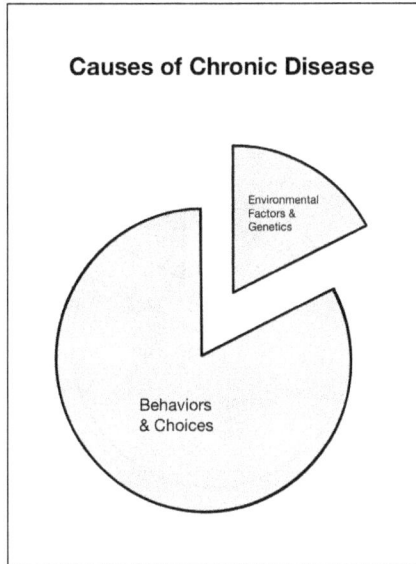

Causes of Chronic Disease

Environmental Factors & Genetics

Behaviors & Choices

Tough Choices

The quality of our long-term health is primarily determined by the quality of our life choices.

Changing behavior is about choosing healthier options, and choosing healthier options is difficult because of ambivalence. Part of us wants to change, but part of us doesn't. Part of us enjoys the benefits the unhealthy behavior brings. These meet a need that part of us, usually a subconscious part, does not want to relinquish. When someone attempts to persuade us to change, that part of us resists.

Think about a time when somebody demanded that you change something. How did that make you feel? Was your first thought, "Okay, no problem," or was your first instinct, "Who are you to tell me what to do?"

What if they had approached the situation differently? What if they had asked for your input and encouraged you to be a part of the solution? Would that have changed your attitude?

Effective Behavior Change

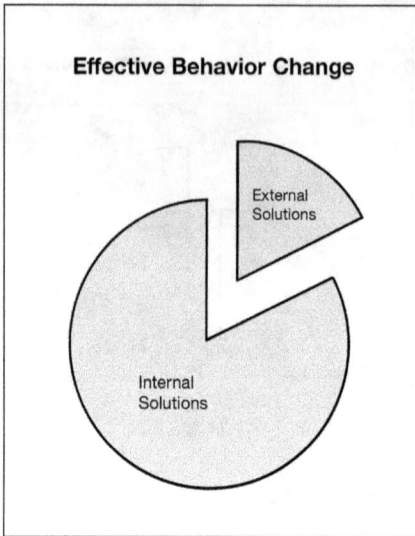

Our current healthcare systems have failed, in part because they haven't been able to help people develop their own solutions. Internally motivating people is a much more laborious and nuanced process. External motivation through persuasion, while less effective, is quick and easy.

Let's look at Ralph. Ralph smokes a pack a day and has done so for 25 years. When he gets anxious or agitated, he uses smoking to calm himself. In addition, when he and his friends socialize they drink a few beers as they smoke. Over the last year or so, Ralph has developed a chronic intermittent cough. His wife nags him until he finally makes an appointment to see his local doctor. Ralph's doctor listens to his lungs and does a breathing test that reveals Ralph has early chronic lung disease. He reminds Ralph of all the other harmful health issues that smoking can cause, like heart disease, cancers and strokes. He tells him to stop smoking and gives him an inhaler to use as needed for his cough and shortness of breath. Ralph struggles to change. Part of him knows smoking is unhealthy, but the other part enjoys smoking. He likes the way it makes him feel, and he is afraid that if he stops he might lose some of his friends. The part of him that wants to continue smoking wins. He is not internally motivated.

What could Ralph's physician have done differently? What if he had slowed down and listened more? What if he had been a little more curious and tried to understand why Ralph wanted to continue smoking? Would that have helped? Maybe, maybe not. The truth is, Ralph will stop when he is ready and not a moment sooner. An internal motivation perspective helps Ralph voice his own reasons for change. An internal motivation perspective listens carefully to Ralph, while paying close attention to the type of language he uses. An internal motivation perspective recognizes that until Ralph begins to talk more about his own desires, abilities, reasons and needs for change, discussing plans for change is premature. Until Ralph is ready, he will most likely resist.

A better healthcare system slows down and listens more closely— two things our current healthcare systems are not incentivized to do. Remember: external solutions, while not very effective, are fast and easy. A better system would help empower people to create internally motivating visions and work with them to design strategies which help them achieve their own goals.

The "experts" who built our current healthcare systems feel that persuasion and education are the primary tools for change, because they believe that people simply don't understand what to do.

Like both Ralph and Carrie, most people already have a basic understanding of what they need to do. They may not understand all the details, but they have a good idea. Their primary struggle is doing what they already know they should do, but may not fully want to do. Effective solutions should focus on helping people fully understand why they do what they do, and then helping them satisfy those needs in healthier ways.

Before we move forward, let's review the difference between the emphasis of our current healthcare systems and a new, more internally motivated system. Traditional healthcare systems agree that chronic disease and unhealthy lifestyles cause the majority of premature deaths; however, the bulk of their attention and resources focus on acute diseases and external factors. If they attempt to modify behavior, it is with externally derived solutions.

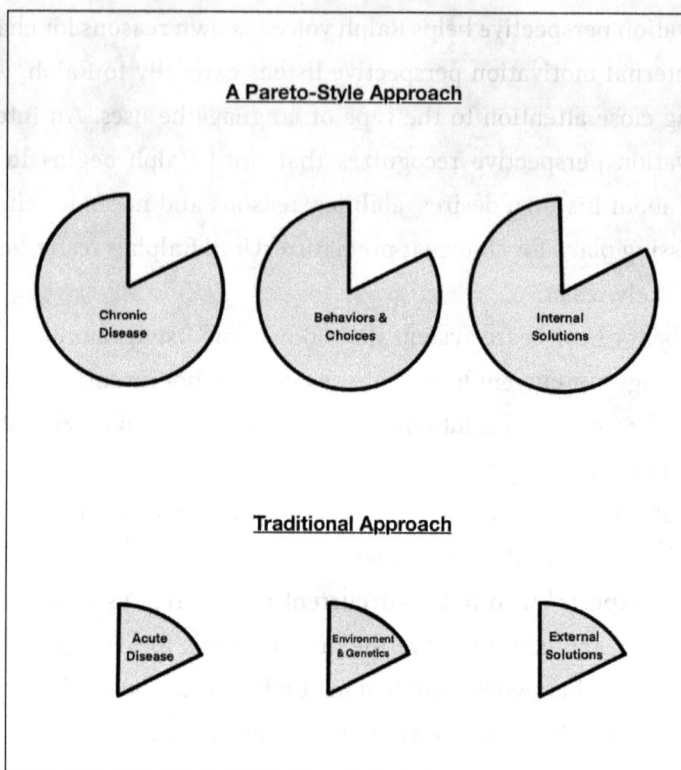

A Pareto-Style Approach

Chronic
Disease

Behaviors &
Choices

Internal
Solutions

Traditional Approach

Acute
Disease

Environment
& Genetics

External
Solutions

A Pareto-style approach concentrates its attention and resources on the big contributors to premature death: chronic disease, behavior change and internally driven solutions. Which sounds more promising to you?

In my work as a physician, it turns out people had been telling me how to motivate them all along. I just wasn't listening. I thought I was, but it wasn't until I gave people enough space to tell me their stories that I began to really hear them. While I had been focused on treating their diseases, people talked to me about their dreams and their visions. They talked to me about how they wanted to walk without pain so they could hike in the mountains. They talked to me about wanting to play on the floor with their grandkids. They talked to me about wanting to dance at their daughter's wedding.

They talked to me about living life. Shrinking disease was important only to the extent that it helped them do something beautiful with their lives.

That's when it hit me. An outline of how to do something much broader than merely treating disease or expanding quality of health was unfolding. Physical health is one thread interwoven with all the other threads that collectively create our lives. What I was beginning to see was a path that helps us collectively strengthen all these threads. Through this more comprehensive process we can build beautiful lives. Now that is exciting.

Physical health relates to many other aspects of our lives, including our emotions, cognitive and spiritual health, our relationships, our career, and our finances.

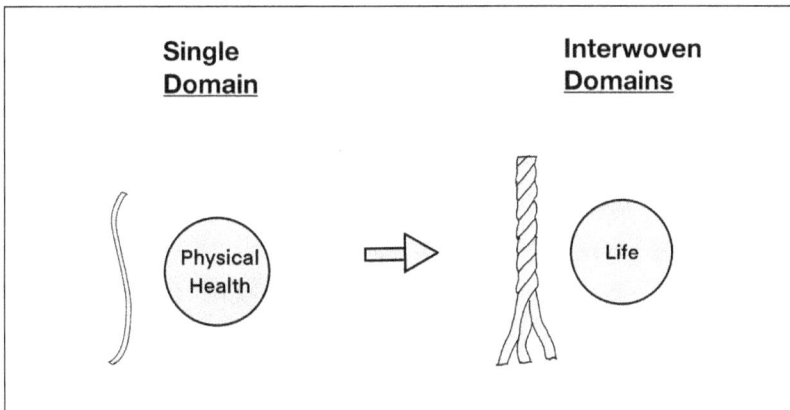

Single Domain — Physical Health → **Interwoven Domains** — Life

While a path was coming into focus, I still had questions about the process:

1. **Who** was going to do it? Who are the responsible parties?

2. **What** is the most important process? The rate-limiting step?

3. **Why** is it even important?

4. **How** do we do it?

This is when I had another revelation. If we could answer these four basic questions effectively, we would have an exciting, comprehensive framework for self-care. I decided to call this model **Empowered Self-Care.**

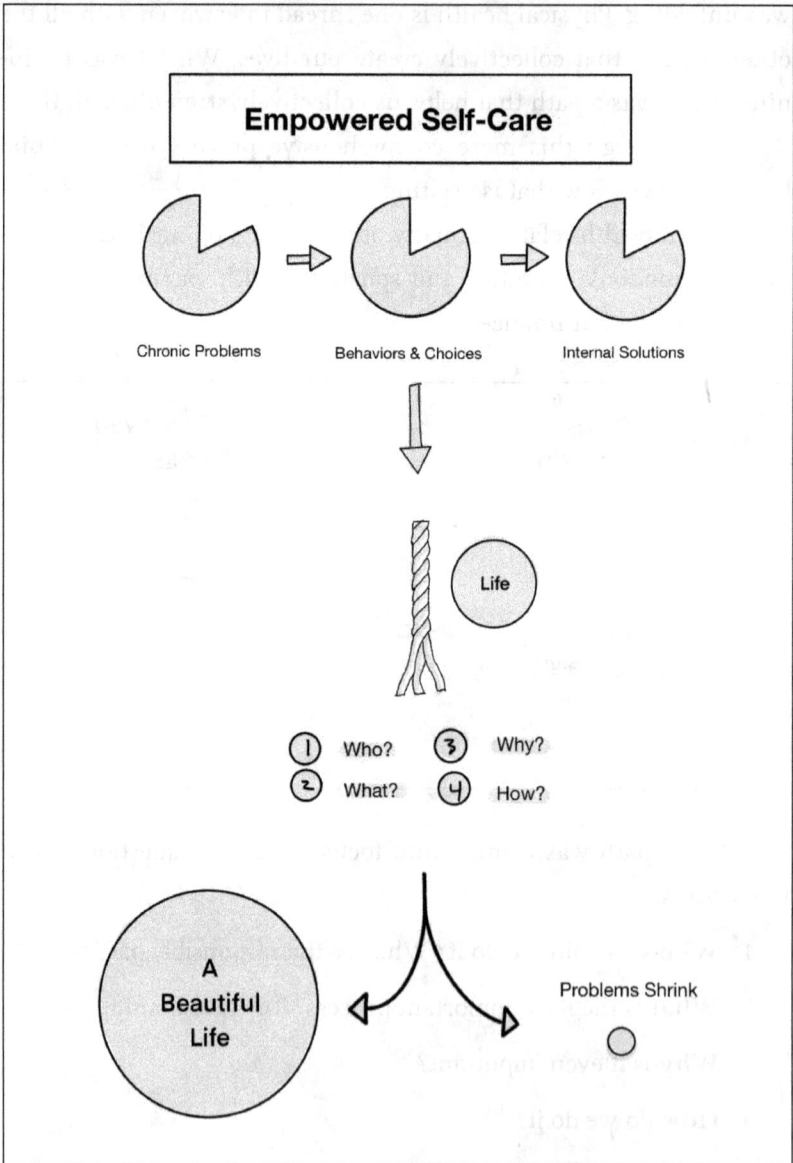

Empowered Self-Care

Chronic Problems → Behaviors & Choices → Internal Solutions

Life

1) Who? 3) Why?

2) What? 4) How?

A Beautiful Life

Problems Shrink

Empowered Self-Care

1. Who?

Empowered Self-Care positions you as your primary care provider, the hero of your own story—**Dr. You.**

Empowered Self-Care embraces a new relationship with expert healthcare providers, one in which you assume active leadership of your personal health. The contrast is similar to the difference between a king and a guide.

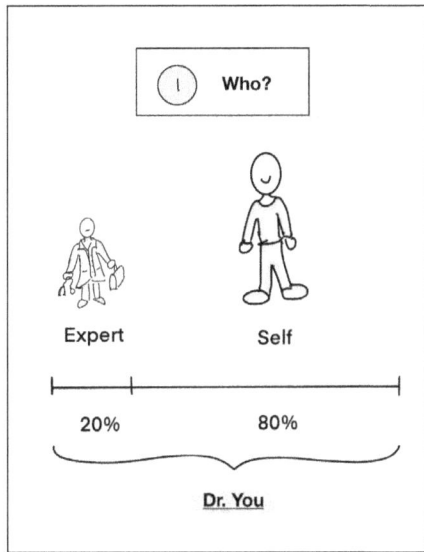

A king issues decrees from afar and expects his subjects to blindly follow. A guide walks alongside a hiker or climber as a fellow journeyman. The guide shares his specialized knowledge while assisting the hiker who does all the difficult work.

As you reassume active leadership of your own care and wellbeing, you effectively become **Dr. You.** In this new role, you don't ignore the experts, nor do they dictate to you what to do. They become your personal board of advisors or compendium of guides.

2. What?

Empowered Self-Care helps you **optimize your brain function.**

It sounds obvious, but you make decisions with your brain, therefore optimizing how well your brain functions will help improve your choices. Optimizing brain function has two parts, **Capacity** and

Power. Experts can help us with both. They can help us sift through the overwhelming quantity of information to find the best, most applicable data. They can also help us develop strategies that improve our ability to apply and use this information.

Even though we have unlimited access to information, the amount the human brain can process at any given moment is limited. This capacity is like a shelf. If the shelf is full and you try to add another book, you'll nudge an existing book off the other side. Most of us understand the bulk of what we need to know to live healthy and fulfilling lives.

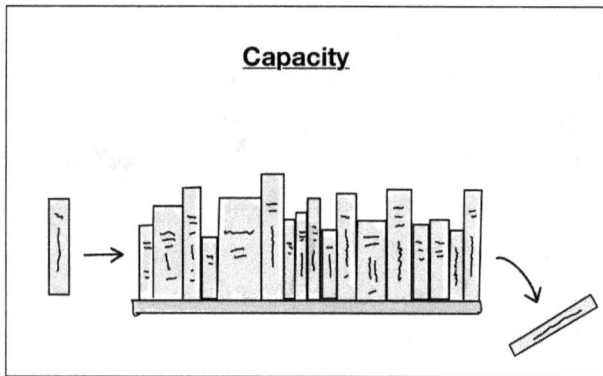

Our mental shelves are filled with excellent information. Twenty percent of the solution may be refining your knowledge base, but **The Big Problem**—80 percent—is applying what we know. I call this **Brain Power.**

Brain Power includes the ability to:

- Plan in consecutive or sequential steps

- Envision distant futures

- Recognize and assign appropriate value (emotions) to people, places, things, and situations

- Engage in creative, divergent thinking

- Attune to spontaneous voices of inspiration or creativity

- Effectively recognize positive opportunities

- Astutely recognize patterns in differing entities or situations

- Bolster motivation for persistent action

While Capacity is limited, Brain Power is expandable. Your biggest potential for growth, therefore, lies in optimizing your brain power.

To explain this better, meet Ned. Ned works for Beautiful Landscaping in the small community of Normalville. Normalville is isolated in a valley surrounded by tall mountains. Ned transports all the flowers, trees, shrubs, dirt, and mulch that his boss uses to create beautiful lawns for the homes and businesses of Normalville. Because Beautiful Landscaping does such a fabulous job, business has grown quickly. Everybody in Normalville wants Beautiful Landscaping to do their landscaping. Running the only truck and trailer for Beautiful Landscaping, Ned struggles to keep up with the demand.

Recently word spread to Distantville, a larger community on the other side of the mountain range, that Beautiful Landscaping does charming and creative work. Ned's boss has accepted a new job in Distantville and has asked Ned to transport the materials for that job which starts in a week.

Ned loads his trailer and heads up the mountain pass. Usually Ned has no difficulty in the flat valley of Normalville, but as he drives up the challenging mountain slope, his truck struggles. Despite driving slowly, his transmission and engine begin to overheat. Eventually he is forced to stop and let them cool. Ned realizes that at this pace he will never complete the job in time. He turns around and heads back down the mountain to Normalville.

His trailer has limited capacity. It is the only trailer in town, and there are no other trailer parts in Normalville. His truck is underpowered, but he does have access to extra engine parts, exhaust tubing and suspension parts.

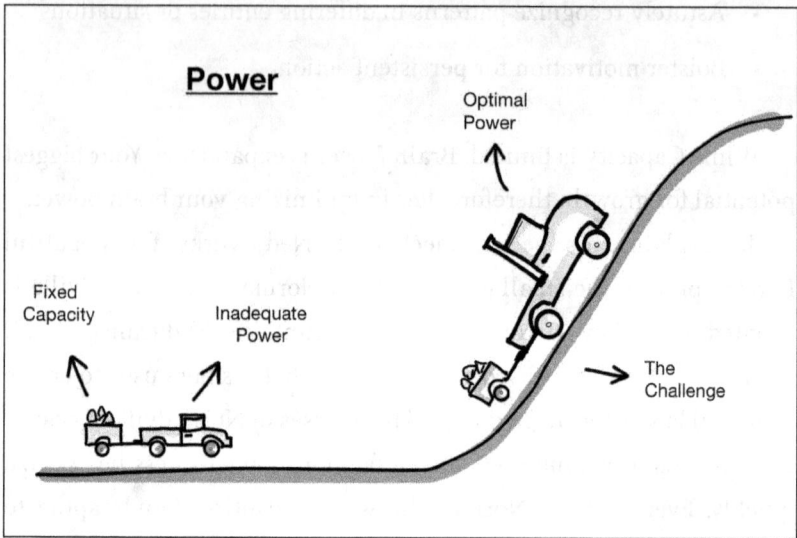

Unsure exactly how he is going to complete his project, Ned begins disassembling his truck, hoping that a solution will appear as he works. A couple of hours into the project, however, Ned feels overwhelmed and as the day progresses, he becomes more and more frustrated. He senses that the more frustrated he becomes, the less effectively he thinks. He finally quits and goes home.

After a good night's rest, he wakes with a new sense of vigor and creativity. As he enters the shop, he runs into Michael the Master Mechanic and asks if he will help. They quickly devise a clever solution. Michael also suggests that Ned use his favorite tool which he promises will make the job a lot easier. With a clear path forward and Michael's time-saving tool, Ned quickly finishes the modifications.

His new, more powerful truck wastes no time scaling the steep mountain pass. Ned finishes the job with three days to spare. His boss is so impressed with Ned's ingenuity that he promotes Ned to Chief Thinking Officer (CTO) and gives him a substantial raise.

Like Ned's trailer, our brains are filled to capacity. We may need to replace some of our outdated information, but developing more powerful ways of thinking is most important. Finding somebody who is just a few steps ahead of us in the process—an expert—can also help us save time and effort. Note that Ned

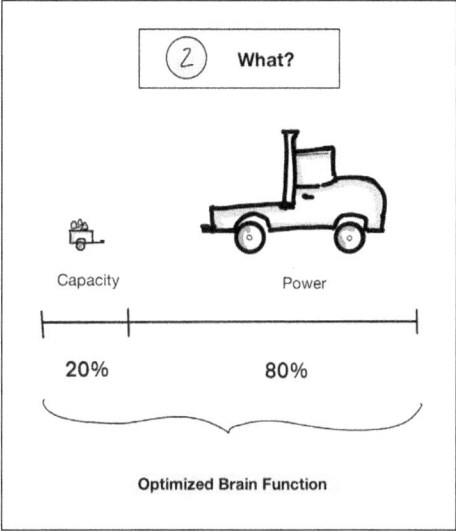

did all the work. His expert guide, Michael the Master Mechanic, simply supported his efforts.

3. Why?

Empowered Self-Care helps you define your strong why, building a beautiful life.

At the intersection of "Who?" and "What?" lies the answer to "Why?": **A Beautiful Life.** Like Goldilocks, it lies between two extremes—not exactly in the middle like the fairytale, but skewed 80 percent to one side. On one end of the spectrum, people rely entirely on an expert, taking no responsibility for their own wellbeing. They have an abundance of information, but no ability to think for themselves. On the other end lie those who accept no help. They are pathologically independent. They quickly become overwhelmed while sifting through a myriad of information and strategies or, even worse, they stop searching when they find overly simplistic, easy-to-understand answers. They not only ignore the insights and wisdom of experts, but they also reject their support.

Building a beautiful life lies 80 percent up the scale toward independence and powerful thinking, but it acknowledges that others can quicken our learning curve and support us when the path becomes difficult.

Each person's why—their Beautiful Life—will be different. It is important you strive to build a life that excites you. It doesn't matter what I think your life should look like. It doesn't matter what your spouse thinks, your pastor or priest thinks or your parents think. What matters is that you can clearly envision a life that excites and motivates you to be the best version of yourself.

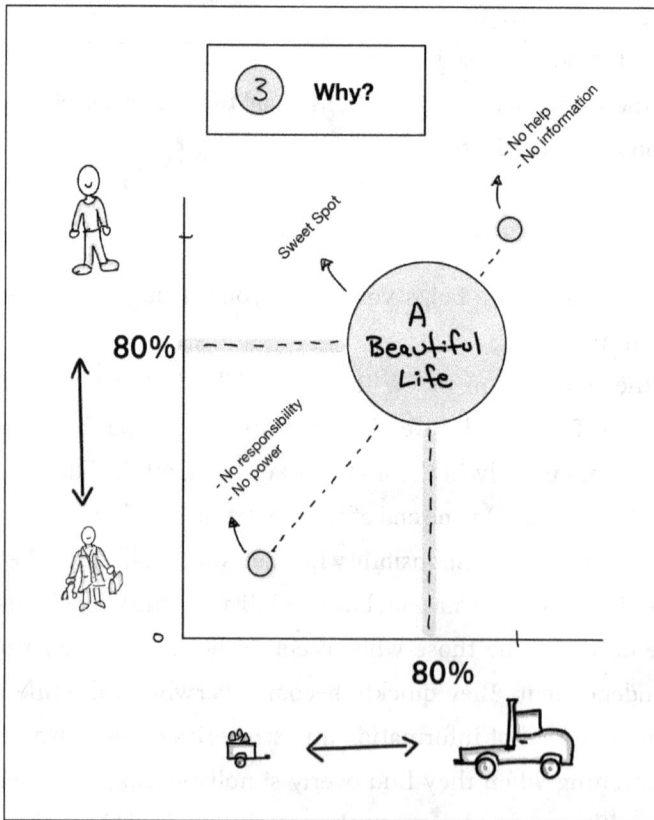

4. How?

Empowered Self-Care is a new powerful tool that helps you build your Beautiful Life.

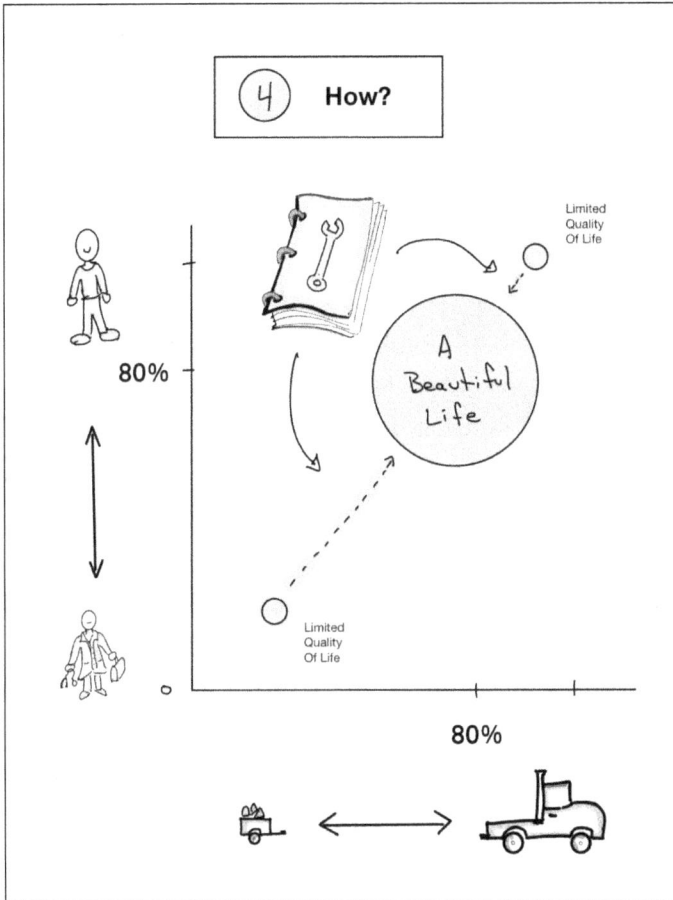

Story has long been used as a way to interpret our experiences and provide a guide for our actions, according to Theodore R. Sarbin, the father of narrative psychology.[7] Many denounce story as a path

---

7   Karl E. Scheibe and Frank J. Barrett, *The Storied Nature of Human Life: The life and work of Theodore R. Sarbin* (Palgrave Macmillan, 2017)

for escapism. Story, however, is not a respite from reality, but a tool that can transport us up a path of discovery. Jordan Peterson, a clinical psychologist in Alberta, Canada, says, "People create their worlds with the tools they have directly at hand. Faulty tools produce faulty results. Repeated use of the same faulty tools produces the same faulty results."[8]

I have attempted to create a tool to help move us along the path of discovery. I call this tool Empowered Self-Care. Empowered Self-Care is a path of self-discovery and self-directing. It is a motivating tool that enhances your natural capacity to take charge of your own life.

Empowered Self-Care changed my life and has helped many others change theirs. I realized that if I wanted something different, it was my responsibility to change, not others or the world around me. If I wanted something different, I needed to become something different or—better yet—I needed to become more of who I was designed to be.

The beautiful life you desire will not come easily. To succeed you will need to maximize every natural resource you have. Empirical evidence and rational thought engage your conscious **Surface Brain,** an important but less powerful region of the human brain. Emotions, feelings, story, and images all engage your more powerful subconscious **Deep Brain.** You must harness both regions to maximize your efficacy. That is the secret strength of Empowered Self-Care. In the following chapters we will discuss how these two divisions of the human brain work and why each of their roles is important.

Empowered Self-Care involves the intentional process of outlining your dreams, goals and solutions into a compelling story, then bringing that story to life. Writing a compelling script helps you focus your attention on what is **Most Important.** It helps you create a clear, concise, unambiguous path for building your beautiful life. We'll discuss

---

8   Jordan Peterson, *12 Rules for Life: An Antidote to Chaos* (Random House Canada, 2018)

in detail how to write your Life Plan in Chapter 9, **Aim**, using the best practices from expert storytellers.

Words are the active expression of an
engaged, intelligent brain. You don't really know
something unless you can clearly convert
your ideas and thoughts into words.

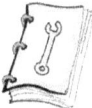

Empowered Self-Care has three phases:

1. Research

2. Plan

3. Do

Empowered Self-Care

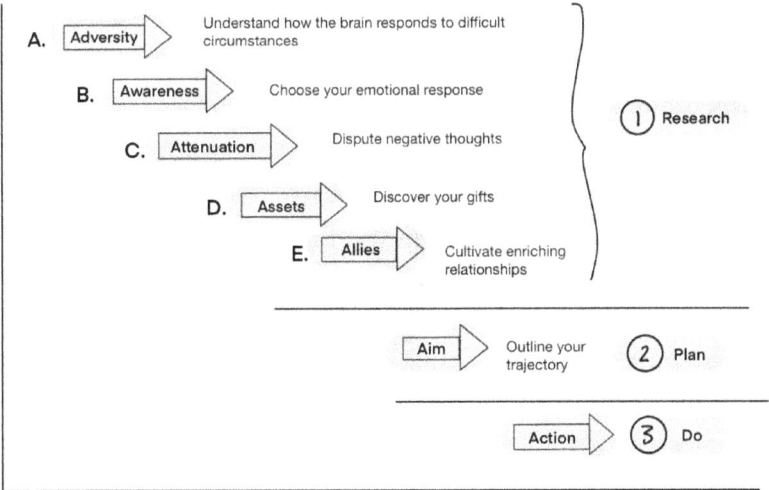

A. Adversity — Understand how the brain responds to difficult circumstances

B. Awareness — Choose your emotional response

C. Attenuation — Dispute negative thoughts

D. Assets — Discover your gifts

E. Allies — Cultivate enriching relationships

① Research

Aim — Outline your trajectory ② Plan

Action — ③ Do

The first phase, **Research,** is where you clarify your preexisting world and put it into words so you can fully understand your journey's starting point. It has five subphases and each will be explained in detail in the following chapters.

a. Inciting event: **Adversity.** Understand how the human brain responds to difficult circumstances. **Chapter 2.**

b. Emotional state: **Awareness.** Learn how to recognize, embrace and choose your emotional responses. **Chapter 3.**

c. Background thoughts: **Attenuation.** Learn to recognize and dispute automatic negative thoughts. **Chapter 4.**

d. Strengths: **Assets.** Discover your natural strengths and gifts. **Chapter 5.**

e. Surroundings: **Allies.** Cultivate enriching relationships and environments. **Chapter 6.**

The second phase, **Plan,** is where you write out your desired trajectory. This is where you **Aim** big and small. Think of this as a flexible map that guides you, but leaves room for alternate paths as opportunities present themselves. **Chapter 7.**

The third and final phase, **Do,** is the most important. Unless you take **Action**, your plans and visions are meaningless. Bring your plan to life by acting it out on the biggest stage, the one called life. This exciting plan will not only help you find meaning and fulfillment, but your treasured story will become your gift to the world. We need you to bring that story to life. This is a summary of the entire process, including some concrete practical steps you can take to initiate your journey. **Chapter 8.**

In a story, after the Inciting Event, the protagonist faces progressive complications which coalesce in the most important point of the climactic scene—the crisis point. Here the protagonist must choose between two difficult options. Should I continue doing the same thing or choose a different path? Should I hold on or let go?

If you do the work, your story will reach a similar point. Are you going to continue doing the same thing or are you going to take a risk and try a new path? Are you going to hold on to your old ways of doing things or let go?

Written correctly, the protagonist grows and transcends, metamorphosing into a different person by the end of the story—and so can you.

Let's return to Carrie's story. Carrie initially comes to visit me feeling defeated. My first visit with her lasts about an hour. Along with reviewing her medical history, we spend a lot of time talking about what is important to her and what she wants me to help her achieve. Over the next several visits, it becomes clear that Carrie is using food and inactivity as a way of coping with work-related stress.

Carrie owns a small clothes-cleaning business that has struggled. Between trying to pay bills, meet payroll and deal with constant personnel issues, Carrie is burning out. When she gets home, all she wants to do is sit on the couch, watch TV, drink a couple of glasses of wine, and eat. She knows that she needs to exercise more, drink less and eat more healthily, but she's not willing to abandon her current ways of relaxing because that's how she unwinds. She's afraid that if she gives them up, she won't be able to deal with the stress of work.

The answer to controlling Carrie's diabetes is not treating her with more medication, and it's not repeatedly telling her to do what she already knows to do—eat better, drink less and exercise more. Carrie needs to change her work environment and learn healthier tools to cope with her stress. Only then will she release her need for inactivity and excess calories. Carrie needs a compelling vision to propel her into action, and only she can create that.

Over the next several weeks, we explore her unique strengths, discover how she emotionally responds to adversity, teach her how to identify and dispute her self-limiting beliefs, and clarify her goals and dreams. She writes all this down in a document. With a clear path forward, Carrie begins to feel empowered and take back control of her life. She still struggles, but today Carrie is in a much better place. She walks for forty-five minutes most days of the week. She has shifted to a more plant-based diet, and has lost twenty-five pounds. Even better, her glucose is now well controlled without any medication.

We all want to be healthy, to feel energetic, to be happy and content, to know that our lives matter. We all can point to areas in our life that we want to—or need to—change so that we can grow. Most of us even know what we should do, but for some reason we just can't seem to do it. Like Carrie, along the way we become frustrated and quit trying.

- Maybe you want to lose weight.

- Maybe you want to become more physically fit.

- Maybe you want to stop smoking.

- Maybe you drink too much alcohol.

- Maybe your relationship with your spouse or another loved one is in trouble.

- Maybe you feel stuck in a dead-end job.

- Maybe life feels overwhelming.

Whatever your struggle, chances are you've reached out to an "expert" for help, maybe even your primary care physician, yet you find yourself still struggling with the same issues. Does that sound familiar?

This book incorporates the findings of many scientific studies, but it is not an academic tome. Rather, it is a manifesto based on my years of experience as a practicing internist and my own search for solutions. It is my invitation to you to look at your health from a different, broader, more exciting perspective.

You need a doctor who cares not only about your physical health, but about helping you build something more meaningful and beautiful with your life. As you change, you'll also change the way people see the world and what they believe they can achieve with their own lives. That is exciting, and the only "doctor" that can help you do that is you—**Dr. You.**

Summary

Most of us know what to do. The problem we all face is that we don't do it. Don't feel bad. This is not a new problem. Even the apostle Paul, one of history's most influential "self-help" writers, had the same difficulty. We all struggle. In the words of Jim Rohn, "What's simple to do is also simple not to do."[9]

Dr. You provides you with a set of core principles you can use to create the better version of yourself you have always desired. It is not a recipe or a specific plan, rather it is an attempt to give you a set of practical tools and a structure to help you clearly define your unique path forward. It is not an attempt for me as a doctor to "heal" you. You must do that yourself. Empowered Self-Care, however, provides you with new and exciting tools for care.

Your path forward will likely not be linear, and you should not feel that these steps need to be followed directly. I started my journey by writing my life plan before I began my research phase. After I learned more about myself, I updated and rewrote my life plan. For example, you may consider reading Chapter 2 on how our subconscious hidden agendas thwart our best logical plans to change. After that, skip to

---

9   Darren Hardy, *The Compound Effect: Jumpstart Your Income, Your Life, Your Success* (Da Capo Press, 2010).

any chapter that resonates with you the most. The important thing is to do what works for you.

If you are frustrated with the paternalistic, dictatorial attitude of many of today's experts and are seeking guidance for a richer and more meaningful life, *Dr. You* is the book for you.

You can find more resources and information at www.DrYou.org.

Here's to your journey!

David W. Ball, MD

CHAPTER 1

Awakening — The Crash

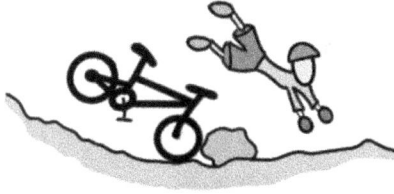

I thought: my crash ended my ability to maintain a healthy lifestyle.

In reality: it opened a door to an even healthier
and beautiful way of living.

---

*"The one who falls and gets up is stronger than the one who never tried.
Do not fear failure but rather fear not trying."*[10]

"The only real mistake is the one from which we learn nothing."[11]

---

10   Paulo Coelho, *The Alchemist* (Harper One, 1988).

11   Henry Ford, AZQuotes.com, Wind and Fly LTD, 2022, https://www.azquotes.com/quote/522550.

The night air was cool and dry as a couple of friends and I unloaded our mountain bikes at Blackjack Turnaround in Tyler State Park. Often we'd see a camper or two here, but not this night. Tonight was unusually quiet and dark. The moon decided not to show itself, so we all fumbled in the dark trying to organize our gear.

I love mountain biking at night. In Tyler, Texas, we don't have access to a lot of trails, so I have ridden the twelve miles at Tyler State Park hundreds of times. I have every little root, rock, branch, and turn along the trail memorized. Riding at night under the confines of our narrow headlamps focuses my perspective and in doing so transforms the experience into something new and refreshing. Because few people ride at this time of night, we traverse the trail backward as well. This helps break the routine even more.

This night had the makings of a great ride. Two of my best riding buddies joined me.

It had been a typical day at work. I am an Internal Medicine physician and at the time had active hospital and outpatient clinic practices. My typical day started early as I made my way to the hospital and rounded on patients by 6:00 a.m. After finishing rounds, I headed to my clinic to review the daily schedule. As with most days, my clinic schedule was divided into back-to-back fifteen-minute appointments. During my lunch break, I grabbed something to eat on the run and headed back to the hospital to follow up on any loose ends from the morning. My afternoon clinic was a repeat of the nonstop morning clinic.

I was living my childhood dream of practicing medicine, yet for the last few years the frantic pace had become increasingly stressful. My clinic schedule had grown tighter and tighter with no margin to catch my breath. If I was lucky, I spent seven or eight minutes with patients. The remainder of the allotted fifteen minutes I spent recording documentation for insurance companies and medical malpractice protection. Little of this is necessary for good patient care, but it is the game we physicians pay to appease the medical gods.

When I talk to businessmen, they describe scheduling time to prepare for each of their daily meetings, and most will have no more than a handful of meetings to prepare for daily. Most primary care physicians have 25-30 "meetings" a day (otherwise known as office visits) crammed into their schedule as tightly as possible. Finding time to whisk away to the bathroom is difficult, much less reviewing anything in preparation for each patient.

I consoled myself by justifying that this busyness must correlate to the degree of impact I was making, but in the recesses of my mind I felt my frustration level building. I knew that I was capable of more and that 7-8 minutes of face-to-face time with patients who have complicated medical histories was not acceptable. I felt not only my own resentment, but also the growing frustrations of patients.

Now at the trailhead, I slipped into the woods and left the clinical world behind. The night air was cool so I zipped my jacket, knowing that within 15-20 minutes I would need to open it again as I warmed up. My body loosened and relaxed as we set off. My breathing settled into a steady, comfortable rhythm and I felt my nerves calming. At this point in the ride, conversations stopped as each of us settled into the steady cadence of churning pedals.

Unlike road cycling, mountain biking requires more riding skill and greater concentration. At a slow pace you can mentally zone out, but at the edge of your capability, obstacles approach at an alarming speed. You find yourself constantly engaging the environment, negotiating turns, jumping over ledges, and plotting the smoothest line between and over roots and rocks. As your speed increases, the skill required grows not linearly, but logarithmically. As such, my mental functions were focused solely on the task at hand. Darkness only enhanced that. I found this focus soothing because it immersed me fully. Nothing else vied for my attention.

My riding buddies' skill set matched my own. Our natural competitive spirit always kicked in and our rides together were faster than our solo rides. Tonight was no exception. My legs were burning as we climbed steep switchbacks and I could feel my rear tire slide as we flung ourselves through turns. I was in my element. The cares of the outside world had slipped away.

I felt strong. I was riding with good friends, and my body felt nimble and fast. I was in my mid-thirties, yet could easily outride kids much younger than me. I was in the best shape of my life. I found myself setting the pace at the front of the group. Your energy level is dependent on several factors: quantity of sleep, intensity of previous work schedule, calories consumed, and stress levels. On rides when you struggle because of a bad combination of these things, you find yourself working extra hard to just stay with the pack.

Then it happened. We were descending a switchback that I had maneuvered through a thousand times before. The corner is a little sandy, with rocks lining the sides at the apex. As I approached it, I realized I was going too fast. I tried to alter my course, but two trees blocked the exit and it was too late to scrub off enough speed. As I entered the apex, my back tire caught the loose sand and slid out from under me. I crashed hard, but not nearly as hard as many other times. My pride was hurt more than anything, I thought.

As I gathered my bike and lifted myself out of the leaves and rocks, I noticed a sharp pain in my left knee. It was not excruciating, but the area was already swollen and bruised. We were about halfway through the ride and the only way back was to proceed forward, so I hopped back on my bike. Something was wrong, however. Every time I applied pressure to the pedal, I experienced a searing, burning sensation through the upper side of my left kneecap. I completed the ride, but struggled the rest of the way.

When we got back to the truck, I examined my knee. My ACL, medial and lateral collateral ligaments, and meniscus were all intact.

No bones were broken. It wasn't a problem a little rest, elevation and ice couldn't fix. The following week I didn't ride, which was extremely difficult. I had worked so hard to build my speed and fitness. I could feel it dissolving. A week later, I jumped on the bike expecting to bounce back, but I still couldn't ride. I started out strong, but after about thirty minutes the searing pain returned.

This continued for the next two years. I underwent months of physical therapy and injections, as well as two surgeries. Nothing worked. It turns out I sustained an odd injury. When I crashed, the upper edge of my left kneecap impacted a rock, tearing a portion of the insertion site of the quadriceps tendon. I had fallen many times before, sometimes resulting in broken bones, including my collarbone, my wrist, a couple of ribs and my leg. I had recovered from these more intense injuries, but I wasn't bouncing back from this one. The tear healed, but I developed a chronic nagging tendonitis at the site of the injury. This injury has ended the careers of a few professional cyclists. My cycling days were over.

That may not seem like a big deal to many, but cycling was not only my way of keeping fit, it was part of my identity. More importantly, it was the primary method I used to cope with stress. With the loss of all these things, I became clinically depressed.

Pressure in my medical practice continued to mount with an ever-increasing workload. Electronic medical records were initially sold to physicians as a way of improving efficiency. This had the opposite effect and at the same time, insurance companies increased documentation requirements for reimbursement. I already felt like my time with patients was compromised, and this compounded the problem. I worked longer and harder to try to keep up. With no effective tools to cope, my stress levels were rising overwhelmingly.

My perfectionism and competitive nature needed an outlet. I have a tendency to push my capabilities to their limits; this followed me into car racing. It made me fast, but unpredictable. I racked up a number of crashes. None of them were very serious, but my racing partner and best friend Mike had to share in the expense of all the body repair costs I incurred.

I loved the adrenaline rush of the speed and competition. I loved the satisfaction of mastering new skills and the focus required. On the racetrack, like on the biking trail, I thought about nothing else but maximizing my speed and staying alive.

I was back—or so I thought. Like cycling, car racing provided an outlet, but I could only do it once a month. What about every other day? I couldn't just jump in my car and blaze down my local street or country roads at 160 mph. I needed a channel for my stress I could immerse myself in more frequently.

Flying was my next choice. Despite the similarities, I didn't see the trend that was forming. My local airport is just a few miles from my house, so I quickly found myself flying consistently three days a week. The problem with flying is that it is even more expensive than racing cars and a lot more expensive than racing bicycles. It also required a lot of time away from my family. I was already working 60-70 hours a week, and now I was flying three days more on top of that.

Remember my tendency to push the limits of my capabilities and my history with mountain bike and car crashes? Joe, another good friend and fellow pilot, nicknamed me The Death Star. I couldn't afford to buy a plane, so I rented one. The problem with that is you never know how other people treat the plane. As such, I experienced more mechanical issues in the short time I had been flying than Joe had experienced in thirty years. I didn't let that deter me, and continued to fly. I didn't realize it at the time, but I was using immersion and thrill-seeking as a distraction to help me cope with the stress and frustration of my work life.

After experiencing engine trouble while flying over Houston— there are no good places to set a plane down over a major city—and having the same thing happen on takeoff from a local airport, I realized that I was going to get myself killed. In addition to that, my work schedule and my flying schedule had become unsustainable. My personal life was suffering. I was spending the majority of my time and focus on work and then trying to distract myself from the repercussions. I was spending little quantity or quality time with my wife and kids.

Now what? I realized that I had an addiction to busyness. I found self-worth in being busy. After all, if I'm busy I must be important. I must be needed. Busyness was killing me, and none of my coping strategies were sustainable or healthy.

Stripped of these, I was forced to face the source of my stress. I finally admitted that I felt a need to prove myself, a need to feel worthy through achievement. I had spent a lifetime trying to prove to myself and the world through academic and social success that I was enough. I had allowed a dark, hypercritical, perfectionistic voice to drive me to become what on the outside appeared to be the definition of success. On the inside however, that dark voice had robbed me of a much kinder, softer voice—the voice that had been quietly telling me all along, "You are already enough."

I was embarrassed of what I had become. I was supposed to be a healer and I couldn't even keep myself healthy. I had been drawn to medicine because of a desire to help others. As a child, I watched my father spend time with his patients in the hospital and during house calls. I had seen first-hand what medicine could be and was supposed to be. I became a physician to be part of a solution, but instead I was part of the problem.

In 2017, I walked away from my lucrative, traditional, fee-for-service practice to start a more patient-centered model. This model slows down and emphasizes relationships. This practice embodies the empowered self-care model by shifting the focus from an external force that heals (i.e. a physician simply dispensing medicine) to a more internal-driven process.

I wish I could say I came to this revelation out of some noble, innate calling. The truth is that my injury left me with no choice. I couldn't proceed as usual. I tried my best to formulate similar alternatives, but nothing else worked. I was lucky. I was forced out of my unhealthy coping patterns because of dumb luck: a simple mountain bike crash one night. It's ironic that adversity on a dark trail shed light toward a healthier, more fulfilling path.

We all have unhealthy coping strategies. Some are more socially acceptable, such as overworking, overexercising, overvolunteering or overeating. Others are less so, such as alcohol, drugs or sex. The end result is the same with each: distraction and numbness. As you read through this book, I want you to think of the various strategies you use to cope with stress. How healthy are they? Do they help you solve the underlying problem, or do they simply mask it? "Out of sight, out of mind" works for a while, but eventually we all must face the root of our stress, fear and anxiety.

My bike crash felt like one of the worst days of my life. With the benefit of time, however, it became one of the best. Sara, my wife, told me several years later that she was glad it happened. It brought me back to the family.

We have all experienced crashes. Maybe yours didn't involve high-speed mountain bikes or racecars, but I suspect you have had unexpected setbacks. Some of these may have been much more pro-found than mine, such as a diagnosis of cancer or the death of a spouse. Sometimes these setbacks take us by surprise and sometimes they are more predictable. How did you get back up once you found yourself face down in the dirt, bruised and bleeding? Are you still lying on the ground feeling rejected and defeated? What lessons did you learn? Are you still struggling to find meaning in those moments of suffering?

This book is my attempt to share what I have learned—and continue to learn—since my crash. It is an attempt for me to redeem myself and my profession. It is an attempt to help gain your trust and show you that we primary care physicians can do better.

I made a set of bookmarks which look like airline boarding passes. They act as physical reminders for me to intentionally stay engaged in the process of meaningful living and not to default to automatic unhealthy responses. They remind me that Adversity—life's crashes—can automatically pull us into unwanted stories, but we can exit those dark storylines by embracing all six components of the departure Gate 6A: Awareness, Attenuation, Assets, Allies, Aim, and Action.

Arrival: Gate 1A (Adversity)

Adversity is the portal that thrusts you into unwanted stories, but it also starts your journey of growth and healing. You can experience growth without adversity, but adversity is often the nidus that forces you to face your problems. Think of *Alice in Wonderland* where Alice falls down the rabbit hole or *The Wizard of Oz* where Dorothy is whisked away by a tornado. Their journeys, like yours, begins through a portal of Adversity.

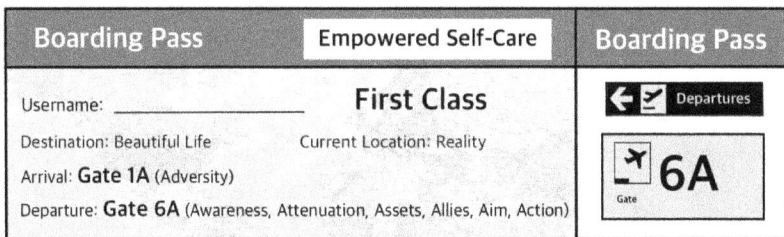

Boarding Pass	Empowered Self-Care	Boarding Pass
Username: _____ **First Class**		← ☑ Departures
Destination: Beautiful Life Current Location: Reality		✈ **6A**
Arrival: **Gate 1A** (Adversity)		Gate
Departure: **Gate 6A** (Awareness, Attenuation, Assets, Allies, Aim, Action)		

Departure: Gate 6A (Awareness, Attenuation, Assets, Allies, Aim, Action)

You exit turmoil and enter the path of meaning when you adopt the six components of Gate 6A. As you acquire and embrace these tools, you will discover that you are able to manage larger and more complex challenges. As you experience success you will develop expanding levels of confidence, motivation, resiliency, and hope. Think of this boarding pass as your golden ticket to living a beautiful life. Depart through **Gate 6A.**

In the next chapter, we will begin to explore the role Adversity plays in shaping automatic beliefs and behaviors.

CHAPTER 2

Adversity — Hidden Obstacles

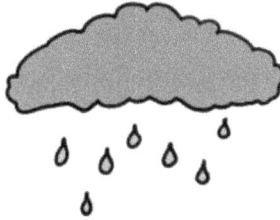

ARRIVAL GATE 1A: Adversity

DEPARTURE GATE 6A: Awareness, Assumptions, Assets,
Allies, Aim, Action

Boarding Pass	Empowered Self-Care	Boarding Pass
Username: _____	**First Class**	← ☑ Departures
Destination: Beautiful Life	Current Location: Reality	✈ 6A
Arrival: **Gate 1A** (Adversity)		Gate
Departure: **Gate 6A** (Awareness, Attenuation, Assets, Allies, Aim, Action)		

Most people think: the majority of their problems
are the result of external adversities.

The truth is: problems often arise because we do not recognize our unconscious, internal needs and do not provide for them in healthy ways.

"If you find a path with no obstacles, it probably doesn't lead anywhere."[12]

"Success is to be measured not so much by the position that one has reached in life as by the obstacles which he has overcome."[13]

After my bike crash, I found myself in an unusual place. When I left my traditional fee-for-service practice I was very physically fit. At my peak I was 9 percent body fat and if asked on any given day I could ride 100+ miles on my bicycle. Then, as often happens, life moved my cheese. My nagging knee injury and the transition into my new practice began to consume more of my time and energy. Slowly, my workouts became shorter and less intense. I began to miss more of them. Even though I never stopped exercising, my lifestyle became more sedentary than it had ever been. Three years later, my jeans felt a bit tighter, none of my trim tailored suits fit and my energy level had dropped.

Slowly and inadvertently, I had "hired" a more sedentary lifestyle to accommodate my waning energy.

Jobs to Be Done

Clayton Christensen was a Harvard business professor who developed the Jobs Theory of economics. In his book *Competing Against Luck* he explains that when we purchase a product or a service we "hire" it to do a particular job. That job-to-be-done is more complex

---

12 Frank A. Clark. (March 28,1860 - April 14, 1936). US Congressman. www.forbes.com/quotes/author/frank-a-clark.

13 Booker T. Washington. (April 5, 1856 - November 14,2015). www.brainyquote.com/quotes/booker_t_washington.

than the obvious functional task of the product. He defines the job-to-be-done as the progress a person is attempting to make in a particular circumstance.

As an example, he shared the story of how his team was hired by a fast food restaurant to help them sell more milkshakes.[14] The company had already spent a lot of money and time surveying their customers to no avail. They asked how they could make their milkshakes better. Do they need to be thicker or chunkier? Do they need to be cheaper? Chocolatier? They tried several of the customers' suggestions, but nothing helped.

Dr. Christensen's team decided to try a different approach. They asked themselves a simple question, "What job are people hiring milkshakes to do?" People don't just buy a milkshake for nutrition. They buy milkshakes for several jobs, but often customers can't express what those jobs are. Christensen's team decided to watch people's behavior first, then ask the job question. They noticed that most milkshakes were sold in two distinct time periods: first thing in the morning and late afternoon.

The early morning crowd hired their milkshakes as a clean, easy-to-consume substitute for breakfast. It worked better than a banana or a bagel because it kept their hunger satisfied all morning. They could consume it with one hand while they were driving. It was less messy than a doughnut. It served as entertainment during their drive, and because they had to suck the thick milkshake through a thin straw, it lasted most of the commute.

The job-to-be-done for the afternoon crowd was much different. Yes, they hired the milkshake for a functional reason—providing nutrition—but the job was more complex than that. The afternoon milkshake buyer was often a parent with kids in tow. As the parent

---

14 Clayton Christensen, Taddy Hall, Karen Dillon, and David s. Duncan, *Competing Against Luck: The Story of Innovation and Customer Choice* (Harper Business, 2016).

ordered meals, the children often asked if they could also get a milk-shake. Parents buying milkshakes in the afternoon were trying to connect with their children, much like buying a toy or spending an afternoon playing baseball.

The morning and afternoon crowds both bought milkshakes for a similar functional need—nutrition—but the social and emotional reasons were different. Armed with this information, the restaurant implemented new strategies to meet these different unspoken needs and successfully increased their sales.

I contend that we hire behaviors and even our different inner personalities—which we will discuss in a later chapter—in similar and more complex ways to meet our unspoken needs.

Dr. Christensen described a fundamental truth of human nature. Often people don't consciously know why they choose one product over another, therefore conclusions based on surveys can be misleading. People's observed behaviors are often more telling because behaviors are a reflection of what people truly believe. Once a business identifies a behavior, they can ask what job a consumer is hiring that behavior to do. That economic question has profound implications for our personal lives as well.

Healthy living follows the same principle as running a successful business. If you force yourself to do things you don't really want to do, you will fail.

What are you hiring your behaviors to do?

The key is to discover the underlying jobs you are hiring a behavior for and help yourself accomplish those deep-seated needs in healthy ways. You must help yourself do the jobs you truthfully want to do, not the things you say you want to do.

Let's look further into eating. As I mentioned in the milkshake story, one job we hire eating for is basic nutrition, but most of us hire food to satisfy other jobs as well. Sometimes it is to solve boredom. Sometimes it is to ease anxiety or to comfort depression. Sometimes it is to provide companionship. Sometimes it is for protection. Sexually abused women sometimes unintentionally hire eating to gain weight. They subconsciously believe that if they gain weight they will become "less attractive" to their abuser, or if they gain size or muscle they can protect themselves more easily.

Questions to ask yourself:

- What are the real underlying needs you have hired your unhealthy behavior to solve?

- What are some healthier solutions you could adapt to solve the true underlying problems?

- How can you design your environment to automatically nudge you in healthier directions?

- How can you place people and systems in your life to help you achieve healthier outcomes?

- What other jobs do you hire this specific unhealthy behavior to do?

Let's take a look at another behavior: spending. We know we should save for the future, but we find it easy to procrastinate. What jobs do we hire spending to do? Sometimes we spend to provide for basic needs like food, clothing and shelter. Sometimes we spend to make ourselves temporarily happy. Sometimes we spend to gain affection. Sometimes we spend to help us feel important and successful.

Maybe the job you hired spending to do is to make yourself feel happy. This might work for a moment, but the effects don't last. So what do we do? We spend more. No matter how much money you have, you can't outspend unhappiness. A better solution is to ask, "If happiness is the job-to-be-done, why am I unhappy?"

As mentioned in the introduction, 80 percent of our runaway healthcare spending is on chronic disease, and 80 percent of chronic disease is the result of unhealthy behavior. Unhealthy behaviors exist because people attempt to meet fundamental needs in the best ways they know how. This is often not conducive for long-term health. Part of us may want to change, but a stronger, often subconscious part, wants to continue the same unhealthy trajectory. Within us rages a war of multiple competing desires.

Medicine has focused its chronic disease policy on simply telling people to do things they don't want to do before walking away. We physicians tell people to exercise and eat better, like they don't already know that. We provide them with simple facts, but don't give them tools or support to accomplish those tasks. Academicians feel that simple education is the solution. Facts are most often not the predominant problem, however. People want to be healthy in the distant future, but providing for an immediate fundamental need or desire that contradicts that is often a much stronger motivator in the present moment. As a result, and as can be predicted, physicians' simplistic advice fails.

Think about an area of life in which you want to become healthier. Do you want to become more physically fit? Do you want more financial security? Do you want more meaningful relationships?

Identify the behaviors that are impeding your progress. That is usually the easy part. The real question is, "Why do we do the things we say we don't want to do?" To help you answer this question, ask another question, the jobs-to-be-done question. What job have you hired those undesired behaviors to accomplish?

Jerry is caught in a spending trap. He has a successful job, but never seems to get ahead. No matter how much he makes, his bills always grow as his income grows. He wants to save more for retirement, but never has enough left over to put into his plan.

Jerry loves fishing. After a long day at work, he grabs his boat and heads out to the lake. He has all the latest gear. He recently bought one of the biggest and fastest bass boats on the market. He knew the payments would be tight, but he stretched the loan out so he could afford them. He also bought the latest multi-thousand-dollar fish finder. His old one worked fine, but this one had more functions.

Sally, his wife, is furious that he bought another fishing gadget. They already couldn't afford his new boat, and now he is spending even more on another "toy." Jerry's fishing—and all of the paraphernalia that goes with it—has become a source of mounting tension. As soon as they get home from work, the arguments begin. Jerry storms off to his corner of the house and Sally to hers. All Jerry can think about is getting out to the lake.

Realizing that they have a problem, Jerry and Sally astutely seek help from a talented marriage counselor. One of the exercises the counselor asks them to do is to identify the things they feel are sources of contention in their relationship. Sally immediately brings up Jerry's spending on fishing equipment. She is furious that he continues to spend on his hobby when they can barely pay their basic bills. Despite her pleas, Jerry continues to spend money they don't have. She feels he is being selfish.

Jerry acknowledges that he spends money when he knows their budget is already tight. The counselor asks Jerry, "What job are you hiring fishing and buying all your fishing gear to do?" At first, Jerry doesn't understand what she means so she asks it another way. "What are you trying to accomplish by going fishing?" His first answer is simply, "I like fishing." But the counselor persists, "But why? What is it about fishing that you enjoy so much?" Jerry admits he feels a lot of pressure at work, and when he gets home the stress worsens because he and Sally are always fighting. He likes to get away from everything. Getting out on the water, where it is quiet and nobody asks him to do anything, is peaceful. He finds that for a few moments he can escape. He also admits when he can't go fishing, he feels better just surfing the internet and looking at fishing gear. Unfortunately when he does, he inevitably buys something.

Jerry and Sally discover that Jerry hires fishing and purchasing fishing gear to do the job of stress relief. Without adequate coping skills and understanding, Jerry feels overwhelmed. He doesn't know how to cope with his job pressures or his escalating marriage problems. Sally's anger only fuels Jerry's sense of overwhelm, driving his unhealthy coping strategy even more. Sally, not knowing how to cope with her mounting frustration, becomes more and more angry. It is a vicious cycle with impending disaster.

Jerry and Sally are not alone in this struggle. Finances are one of the most contentious areas for married couples. Often one or both have hired spending as a way of soothing the stressors of life. Small infrequent "sinful pleasures" like this are not problematic, but when they become the primary means of coping, problems ensue. We must address these root problems.

Asking that simple job-to-be-done question is a good step toward shedding light on your underlying motivations or needs. Sometimes these remain stubbornly hidden in the shadows. When that happens, we need to continue to ask questions.

I like using the "Five Why" technique. In our above example, Jerry asked the first most important question, "What job have I hired fishing and spending on fishing paraphernalia to do?" He discovered, or at least now consciously admitted, that he hired them to help him deal with stress, but why was he stressed?

The Five Why Technique

To help him understand this, his counselor uses the "Five Why" technique to help him discover the source. Let's look at how this works with Jerry.

1. Why are you so stressed? Answer: I feel overwhelmed.

2. Why do you feel overwhelmed? Answer: My boss expects me to do too many things at once. He gives me all this busy work and gives the things I enjoy doing and am good at to somebody else.

3. Why does he give you the busy work and not the things you enjoy doing? Answer: I don't know. I've never said anything to him.

4. Why haven't you said anything? Answer: I was afraid that I would be demoted. Sally and I need the money.

Now we are beginning to get to actionable steps—the real job that needs to be done. After several sessions, Jerry discovers that he feels trapped in the office. He recently accepted a promotion to a managerial position because it pays better. He and Sally need the extra money, but he hates managing people and all the paperwork it requires.

It turns out, he's not very good at being a manager and despite his best efforts to bolster his weaknesses he is performing poorly at his job. He knows it, and his boss lets him know it daily. He is a salesman by nature. He loves outside sales. He is great at sales. He enjoys travel and the challenge.

Jerry's out-of-control spending intensified when he took the promotion. Jerry neither needed more money nor a job he hated. He needed to learn healthier coping skills. Once he did this, his spending dropped, and he returned to the job he was uniquely gifted to do: outside sales.

Like Jerry, by the time you get to your fifth "Why," and maybe sooner, you will discover your own core issues. When you understand the root of your problem, you can develop strategies to solve it. On paper it sounds easy, but in reality it can be difficult, especially when a sense of overwhelm clouds your ability to think clearly.

How can you use the job-to-be-done question to open a path for your own healing? The job-to-be done question is the gate that leads to a path of enlightenment and the journey of empowered self-care. Are you ready to become your own Dr. You?

Let's go back to the beginning of the chapter. What job did I hire a sedentary lifestyle to do? Providing for my family and building a practice were my priorities. I spent most of my non-work time reading and studying how to build a successful business and develop a creative new medical model. If a sedentary lifestyle is something you struggle with, stop now and ask yourself, "What job have I hired sitting on the couch and watching TV to do?"

Inactivity helped me solve my fatigue and stress problems, but only temporarily. I hired a less active lifestyle to give me more energy. I hired a less active lifestyle, sitting on the couch and reading a book, to provide an escape from reality and to help me cope with stress. I felt tired because I was not getting enough sleep, because my diet was not as nutritious as it should have been and because I lost my physical reserves. Being less active temporarily alleviated the symptoms, but it exacerbated the long-term problem. That's the problem with unhealthy behaviors.

Sometimes you will find your difficult emotions are rational and legitimate. Like a traffic light, they draw attention to an area of your life that needs to change. But perhaps circumstances are not going to change anytime soon, or at all. What then? How do you cope with those difficult and painful emotions in a healthy, productive way?

Empowered Self-Care: A Mechanism to Dampen the Negativity Bias

This first step is to take an inventory of your life.

Every year, my team and I perform an extensive physical on each of our patients. Some of the things we do are similar to what your primary care physician does. We listen to their hearts and lungs, examine their thyroid and do a skin review. In addition to that, we measure metabolic rate, check bone density, measure muscle mass, body fat and visceral fat, perform an exercise test, run routine blood tests and advanced cardiac blood tests. This gives us a running baseline of our patients' physical health.

Your overall health, however, depends on the health of all the domains of your life, not just your physical health. I therefore ask our patients to visualize their life as a composite of these different Life Domains. I ask them to divide their life into the 5-10 domains that they think are most important. For example, you may think about faith, family, friends, finances, and fun. My working categories are physical health, emotional health, cognitive health, spiritual health, spouse, children, friends, career, finances, and hobbies. (Figure 2.6) The most important element of the exercise is to list the domains that matter most to you. Write them along the bottom of the blank Dream Assessment Chart in Figure 2.7.

What am I doing today to progress the dream?

DREAM ASSESSMENT										
	Physical Health	Emotional Health	Cognitive Health	Spiritual Health	Career	Finances	Spouse	Children	Friends	Hobbies
10										
9										X
8			X							
7										
6				X						
5										
4	X									
3								X		
2						X				
1										
0										
-1										
-2										
-3								X		
-4										
-5		X		X						
-6							X			
-7										
-8										
-9										
-10										

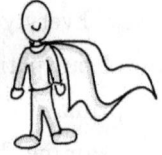

Soaring

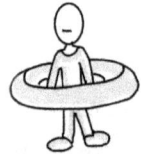

Surviving

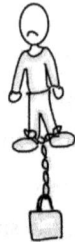

Sinking

(FIGURE 2.6)

Next, subjectively rank your satisfaction in each of these domains on a scale from -10 to +10. Don't think about it too much. I want your initial gut feeling.

What am I doing today to progress the dream?

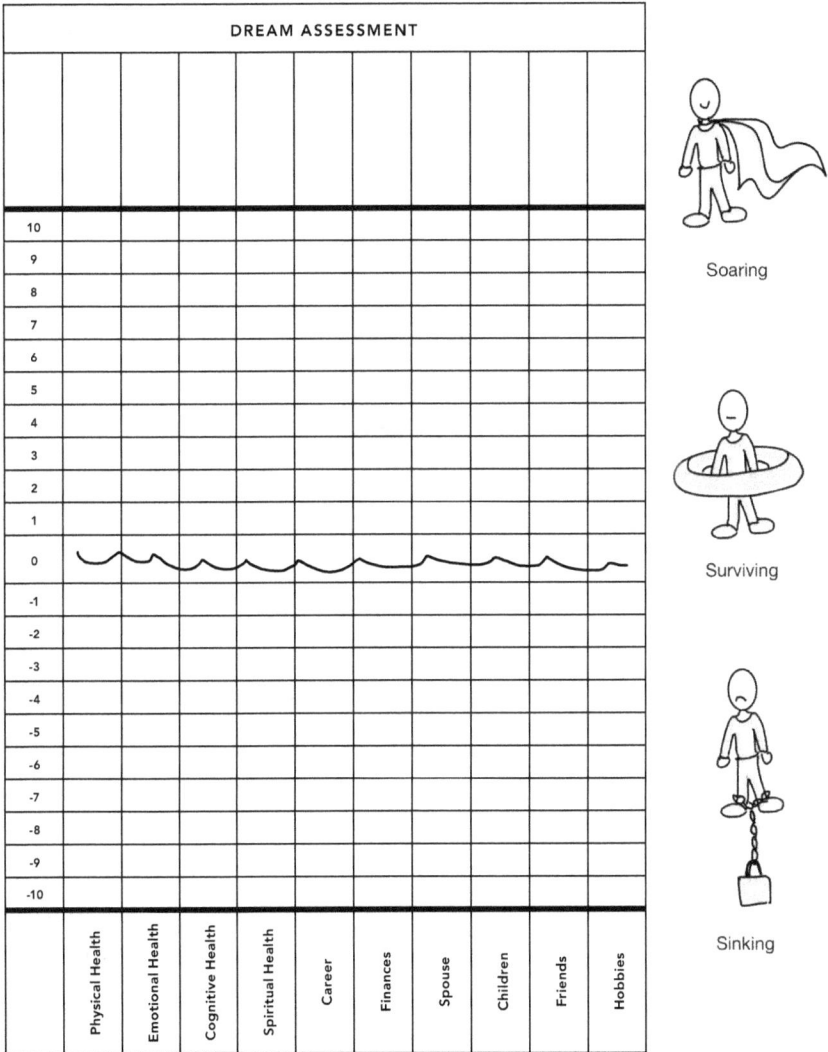

(FIGURE 2.7)

Zero is neutral. You are surviving, but just treading water. At a -10, you feel like you are drowning, sinking into an abyss. At a +10, you're soaring. Here, life is perfect. Not too many of us rank our lives as perfect, and most don't feel like they are being crushed by the weight of the world. Most of us feel like we are in the middle somewhere. But just surviving, just making it from day to day, is not what we long for. Treading water is better than sinking, but we yearn to fly. We dream of a life filled with love, joy, happiness, meaning, and purpose. We long for the fullness and richness of a grand adventure.

Now that your inventory is complete, how does your life look? Are you progressing toward your dream? Do you want to improve any of your domains? What is holding you back? For most of us, ambivalence is the problem. Part of us wants to strive for a better place while, simultaneously, part of us enjoys the benefits of our current state. Unfortunately, the latter often prevails.

What does living a good life mean? What does that look like? Better yet, what does building a beautiful life look like? That sounds more exciting. That sounds like something more worthy of working toward.

Unless you're one of the lucky few who won the genetic lottery and are always happy and optimistic, building a beautiful life will take effort. It will require you to live smarter and more deliberately. You will need to learn new skills and specialized knowledge, and acquire new tools.

Maybe your relationship with your spouse is good, so you ranked it at a +3. Are you satisfied with that or do you want better? Maybe you did well in school, but since then you haven't applied yourself to learn anything meaningful. Maybe you want to learn a musical instrument or a new language, but feel you're too old to start something new.

Modern psychology has much to say about how to enrich the positive side of life. We will discuss this in the chapters on Assets, Allies and Aim. If all your life domains are ranked above the waterline and you are ready to soar to higher levels, you may want to skip to the Assets chapter. Here you will discover a process to uncover and apply your natural giftedness. After this, in Allies, you will learn how to create fertile environments for growth, and in Aim you will learn how to write a powerful actionable plan to help you apply all your new insights.

If Adversity has taken control of your life, you may feel that one or more of your life domains has sunk deep into the abyss. Your attention will likely be consumed by those areas. This is natural. It is part of our designed negativity bias. In the days when life was filled with physical dangers, a bias toward things that could harm us was helpful. In modern times where the most dangerous things we face are often our own feelings, a negativity bias can cause untold issues. If you are stuck in survival mode and fighting unseen enemies, you will have little time and energy to focus on the more pleasurable and productive part of life.

Common solution: Internal healing vs. external blame

Sonja Lyubomirsky is a distinguished professor of psychology and researcher at the University of California, Riverside and the author of *The How of Happiness*. Her research reveals, contrary to what most people think, that external circumstances account for only 10 percent of your happiness. Fifty percent of your happiness is determined by your genetics and 40 percent is directly controlled by your intentional activities. You can't significantly alter most external factors, and your genetics are even less modifiable, but your intentional activities are 100 percent within your control. I find it encouraging that what we choose to do influences our moods in such a significant way.

Your genetics and the environment in which you were raised broadly determine your mood setpoint. Mood setpoint is similar to weight setpoint. Some people are naturally skinny, some muscular and others more plump. Your body tries to maintain your weight within a narrow range, and your brain similarly tries to maintain your mood within your natural range. Your mood setpoint lies on a continuum between pessimism on one end and optimism on the other. Most people's mood setpoints fall in a small range somewhere in the middle. As you engage in pleasurable activities, you move your mood setpoint up the scale within your genetically determined range. Painful experiences have the opposite effect. However, as you will learn in the next chapter, it's a little more complicated than this. Some pleasurable activities have a more sustained mood-lifting effect than others. You will also discover that if you ignore difficult emotions and attempt to compulsively suppress or numb them with simple pleasurable activities, your brain will build a tolerance to those activities. The trick is engaging in activities that sustain happiness while simultaneously allowing yourself to safely experience the discomfort of difficult situations.

Healing ourselves starts with a simple switch in focus. It begins when you stop blaming other people and external situations for your problems and focus on behaviors you can control. You can't control other people; you can control yourself. As you focus on your intentional activities, you can promote healing and initiate the process of becoming a better version of yourself.

Unlike more passive treatment paradigms, Empowered Self-Care calls you to act with intention. You assume the responsibility of becoming your own primary care provider and rely on others in a supportive role as secondary care providers.

The Boarding Pass I introduced in Chapter 1 reminds us of this innate capacity to control our lives. While we may not be able to control when Adversity arrives, we can depart from its stranglehold through the six intentional components of **Gate 6A.** I keep several of these boarding passes in my briefcase to use as bookmarks and to give to other people. They empower me by refocusing my attention on the steps I can take to build a better, more beautiful version of my life. You can also deliberately depart your dark storylines by using these same six techniques. In the next chapter we will introduce the intentional departing step, **Awareness.**

Boarding Pass	Empowered Self-Care	Boarding Pass
Username: _____ **First Class**		← ✓ Departures
Destination: Beautiful Life　　Current Location: Reality		✈ **6A**
Arrival: **Gate 1A** (Adversity)		Gate
Departure: **Gate 6A** (Awareness, Attenuation, Assets, Allies, Aim, Action)		

Summary

1. Your observed behaviors are a better indicator of what you truly believe than what you say.

2. Part of us wants to act in healthy ways, but a stronger part doesn't. You want to be healthy in the distant future, but providing for an immediate need or desire that contradicts that is often a much stronger motivator in the present moment.

3. We often hire unhealthy behaviors to perform certain "jobs" for us.

4. Empowered self-care begins by taking an inventory of your top 5-10 life domains. What do you need to do in each domain to become a better version of yourself?

5. Fifty percent of your happiness is determined by your genetics, 40 percent is determined by your intentional behaviors and only 10 percent is determined by your external circumstances.

Understanding and coping with **Adversity** in healthy, productive ways can be difficult in part because it feels uncomfortable. We don't like discomfort, so we automatically try to make it disappear. We resist. Most often, that occurs through our unhealthy coping mechanisms. The problem is that the discomfort we feel, the strong emotion, is an important signal to which we must learn to pay attention. In the next chapter, **Awareness**, I will discuss how our brains use emotions to communicate with us, and how to process these feelings in constructive ways.

CHAPTER 3

Awareness — Explore Your Emotions

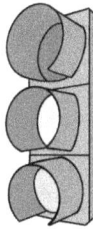

ARRIVAL GATE 1A: Adversity

DEPARTURE GATE 6A: Awareness, Assumptions, Assets, Allies, Aim, Action

Boarding Pass	Empowered Self-Care	Boarding Pass
Username: _____	**First Class**	← ☑ Departures
Destination: Beautiful Life Current Location: Reality		✈ 6A
Arrival: **Gate 1A** (Adversity)		Gate
Departure: **Gate 6A** (Awareness, Attenuation, Assets, Allies, Aim, Action)		

Most people think: that building a beautiful life requires focusing on experiences that make us happy while ignoring those that don't.

The truth is: building a beautiful life requires embracing the full gamut of emotions and experiences, including those we find most difficult.

"What is necessary to change a person is to change his awareness of himself."[15]

As a primary care physician, I have the privilege of walking alongside people during their "best of times" and "worst of times." I am continuously amazed by how well some shoulder the most intense adversities, like the death of a spouse or child, while others crumble under much more modest trials. If prosperity were the solution, you would think that the most rich and powerful among us would prevail, but I have found it to be the opposite. Ordinary people from the humblest of backgrounds often persevere in the most noble ways, while society's most fortunate often wilt in a cocoon of self-absorption.

On the day I first met Stephanie, the tires of her brand new 700 series BMW screeched as she swerved into the parking lot. She walked in with an air of confidence, wearing the latest designer clothing and accessories befitting someone of her social stature. At 38 years old, she was beautiful and wealthy—the picture of success. In the privacy of the exam room, however, her countenance changed.

After introductions and a few cursory comments, I asked how I could help. She immediately shared that none of her other doctors had been able to help her. She had been on pain meds for years and said she didn't like the way they made her feel, but she hadn't found any other way to control her pain. Her lower back constantly hurt, but no surgeon had found anything significant enough to correct. Her chronic recurring migraines hadn't responded to traditional non-narcotic therapies, nor did her fibromyalgia. The only thing that seemed

---

15 Abraham Maslow, https://www.brainyquote.com/quotes/abraham_maslow_132272.

to work was an ever-increasing dose of narcotics. Each escalation of her dose seemed to help for a while, but its effects soon waned, leading to further increased doses. She was taking Oxycodone, Hydrocodone and Lyrica prescribed by three different physicians and filled at four different pharmacies. Along with that, she was taking Adderall for ADD, Xanax for anxiety and Ambien for insomnia. With each additional complaint, a new potentially addictive medication had been added into the already-toxic mix.

Stephanie's wealth was not self-made. She grew up in a prominent wealthy family. Her father was the stereotypical successful, workaholic, emotionally unattached, playboy businessman. Her mother was quite the opposite. A quiet, unassuming woman, she lacked healthy coping skills to meet her own emotional needs, much less those of her children. Stephanie described her mother as a solemn, isolated, depressed person who she vowed never to be like. Both parents were neither physically nor emotionally available and deferred the responsibility of raising Stephanie to her nanny. Her parents' primary means of connection with Stephanie was by buying her things.

In her early teenage years, Stephanie began drinking alcohol and smoking marijuana. By the time she was in high school, she was experimenting with prescription drugs. Constantly in trouble and failing her classes, she was sent to a strict private boarding school, which worsened her sense of isolation.

She eventually graduated high school and was admitted to a small private university, but only after her father made a substantial donation. In college, Stephanie was known more for spending her daddy's money and partying than for her academic discipline. During her sophomore year, she was admitted into a drug rehab program for the first time, but left before completing it. Ultimately, she dropped out of college and married a wealthy man twenty years her senior who could support her spending habits.

Over the next couple of decades, her life continued to spiral further and further out of control. When she walked into my office, she had been married four times, was currently divorced and had been involved in a litany of other failed relationships. Her relationship with her family was strained, and her parents had stopped paying for rehab programs. She was firmly addicted to prescription medications and spending her trust fund, but—in her own words—her pain was still uncontrolled.

When you hear Stephanie's story it's easy to cast stones, but we all have our addictions. Most of them are more socially acceptable, or at least easier to hide. By addictions, I mean anything we use to numb or suppress the difficult emotions we don't want to feel. Often, we employ these addictions subconsciously. We distract ourselves from feeling with social media, inactivity, the internet, shopping, eating, gambling, pornography, sex, work, excessive busyness, smoking or TV. Some of these activities are acceptable in moderation; the problem comes when we use them to satisfy needs that they were never intended to meet and to suppress and numb unwanted emotions.

Dopamine, The Pleasure Hormone

To understand how this works, let's look at one of the key pleasure hormones of the brain—dopamine. Dopamine is a neurotransmitter used by neurons to communicate with each other. When you engage in enjoyable activities, the neurons of the brain's pleasure centers release dopamine. The dopamine released by the end of one neuron crosses the gap, or synapse, between two neurons and then attaches to specially designed docking stations called receptors on the next neuron. Once dopamine attaches to its receptors, a biochemical electrical signal is produced that then travels through the neuron to the next neuron in the chain, and the cycle repeats itself. (Refer to Figure 3.1)

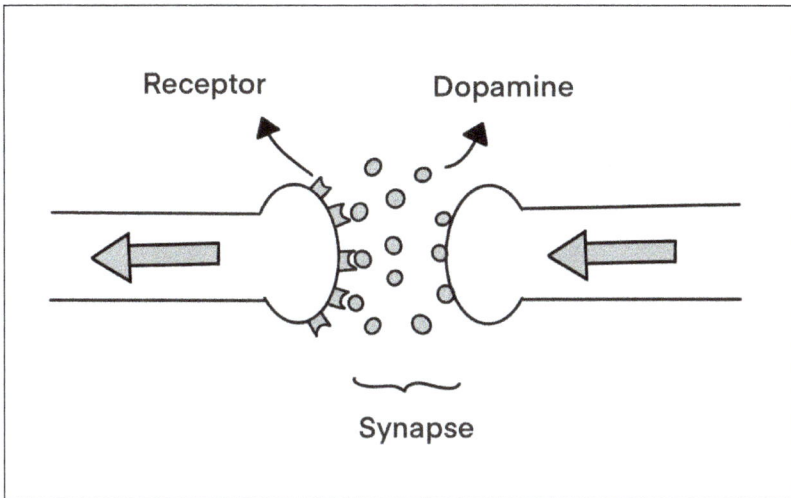

(FIGURE 3.1)

The more intense the pleasurable activity, the greater the amount of dopamine released and the more intense the electrical signal produced by the receptors—up to a point. The human brain prefers to maintain a level of homeostasis, or balance. Each of us is born with an emotional setpoint, or level of happiness that your brain naturally prefers to maintain. Think of your emotional setpoint not as a single point, but as a small range on a larger scale with extreme pessimism/depression on one end and extreme optimism/happiness on the other. Some psychologists refer to this setpoint as your Explanatory Style. We'll discuss more about explanatory style in a later chapter.

If you do something or something happens to you—good or bad—that deviates your mood from your natural setpoint, your brain will eventually bring it back. Think of it this way: if you lose a $100 bill you will be sad for a time, but eventually your mood will drift back to its usual happier state. The same thing happens when you enjoy a mood-lifting experience, like a funny movie. For a short time your mood will be unnaturally elevated, but eventually it will settle back to your setpoint. Homeostasis has survival benefits. As your mood settles, you remember what it feels like to lose and what it feels like to experience pleasure. With those learned experiences now programmed strongly in your memory, you seek to avoid loss experiences and pursue pleasure experiences.

Emotional homeostasis is particularly important in times of scarcity or turmoil. It helps us recover from disappointment while making us stay vigilant and motivated to pursue better states of living. The system does have its downsides, however, especially during times of plenty. When simple pleasures are easily available and our natural instinct is to seek them out, we have a tendency to over consume. In times of scarcity, overconsumption doesn't occur because we don't have ready access to these pleasures.

With chronic overconsumption of pleasurable activities, dopamine is excessively released and your brain becomes overstimulated. In an attempt to return your emotional state to your natural setpoint, your brain reduces the amount of dopamine released into the synapses and downregulates the number of receptors available to receive it. (Refer to Figure 3.2) Now your preferred addictive behavior doesn't produce as much pleasure, thus requiring more of the behavior to achieve the same effect. Eventually, you require extreme levels of stimulation just to feel normal or balanced. It is a vicious trap that we all can fall into.

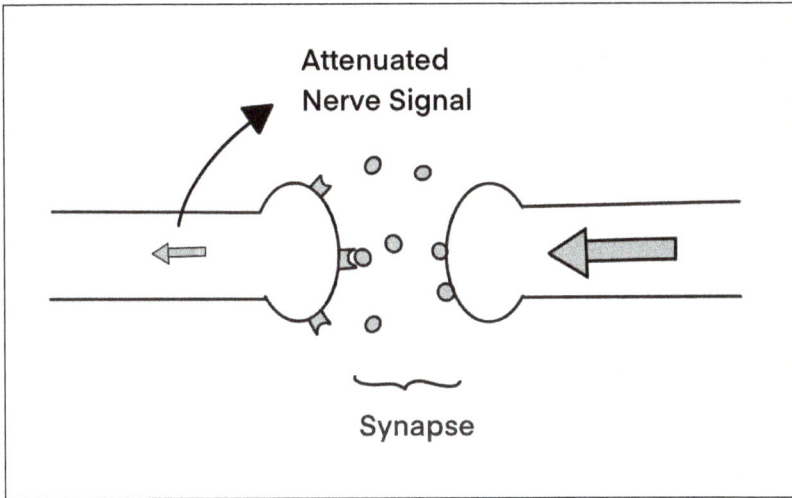

Attenuated
Nerve Signal

Synapse

(FIGURE 3.2)

The key to preventing this or returning to a healthy, balanced emotional state is to first stop compulsively stimulating the system with your preferred addictive behaviors. This encourages the brain to upregulate or increase the number of dopamine receptors and release larger amounts of dopamine in response to more ordinary behaviors. In the short-term, while your brain is readjusting, dopamine levels drop more quickly than your brain's ability to upregulate the receptors, therefore you will feel worse before you begin to feel better. This means you must allow yourself to feel the discomfort of difficult emotions and sensations that you have been avoiding. The paradox of healthy emotional regulation is that in order to keep pain in check, you must allow yourself to feel it first. Suppressing it only intensifies it.

Traffic Signal of Emotions

Awareness is the process of allowing yourself to feel the full gamut of emotions without judgment. Only in the safety of this non-judgmental attitude can you clearly understand what your difficult emotions are trying to tell you. Positive, happy emotions are easy to under-stand, but why should anyone experience negative, difficult feelings?

Emotions assign value, or valence, to people, places, things, and circumstances. Without this system of valence, like Spock in *Star Trek,* you would process all situations and circumstances equally. Charles Darwin proposed that the fundamental purpose of emotions is to initiate movement that will restore the organism to safety and physical equilibrium.[16] The ability to interpret your emotions and the emotions of others is critical to functioning cohesively as part of a larger society.

I like to think of emotions as traffic signals. "Negative," or what I will refer to as "Strong" or "Difficult" emotions, are not negative at all. All emotions are intrinsically good and helpful. Strong emo-tions serve as warnings, like red lights. Red lights at intersections aren't bad. They're protective. They tell us to slow down, stop and pay attention. These emotions often emerge from our subconscious, or Deep Brain. Similarly, think of positive emotions as green lights. They tell us that all is good and safe to proceed. Intersections with single-colored traffic signals would be dangerous to enter or leave us with no option to proceed forward. Life with only one shade of emo-tion would be similarly difficult to navigate.

Also, like traffic signals, emotions are helpful only when you pay attention to them, know how to interpret them and then use that information to change your behavior. Catastrophes ensue when you ignore the signals, don't understand how to interpret them and don't alter your behavior.

---

16 Bessel Van Der Kolk, *The Body Keeps the Score: Brain, Mind, and Body In the Healing of Trauma* (Penguin Books, 2014).

Resisting vs. Awareness

When difficult emotions feel dangerous, scary, overwhelming or threatening, the automatic tendency is to resist them and prevent yourself from experiencing them. Unfortunately, this leaves you blind to their warnings. Awareness, on the other hand, involves allowing yourself to experience difficult emotions with curiosity and compassion. Resisting, as Kristin Neff, PhD, a mindfulness compassion researcher explains, is a slippery slope. When we initially encounter difficult emotions, people tell themselves, "I don't like this feeling." It then becomes, "I don't want to feel this." Judgment then subtly slips in as a "should" statement: "I shouldn't feel this way." This becomes, "Something is wrong with me for feeling this way." Finally, as ruminations build, we ensnare ourselves in a prison of shame: "I am bad."

Neff says that we progress through five stages, represented by the acronym RETAB, as we learn to relate to our difficult emotions in healthier ways:

Resist

Explore

Tolerate

Accept

Befriend

Initially we **resist** difficult emotions. As noted earlier, we don't like the uncomfortable sensations they produce in our bodies. We don't want to feel them. They threaten our sense of security.

Once we have calmed our bodies, a helpful next step is to adopt the curious mindset of an explorer or researcher. Curiosity has no agenda but to discover hidden truth, whatever that truth may be. Freed from a set outcome, we now can **explore** our emotions from a safe distance. Simple repeated exposure naturally leads to **tolerance.** With tolerance, we begin to understand where our deep emotions originate and what they are trying to accomplish. We begin to **accept** them for what they are. Acceptance yields the insight that difficult emotions represent something good and beautiful about ourselves. In their own way, our difficult inner emotions try to protect us. Understanding their sacrificial, servant nature helps us feel compassion toward them. With compassion, we can **befriend** them for their efforts to serve us.

A Choir of Emotions

Another way to picture the role of emotions is as individual singers in a choir. Each choir member is assigned a specific part to sing. When every member sings their part in perfect harmony, the result is a powerful and beautiful unified effort. If someone sings out of tune, however, their efforts stand out and automatically draw your attention to the problem. Strong emotions are similar. They focus your attention and motivate you to change something. Their asynchronous activity intentionally produces discord that your internal leader, your conscious or Surface Brain, naturally wants to resolve. The goal is not to suppress or ignore the out-of-tune singer/strong emotion. The goal is to identify the source of the problem and correct it.

Both the Surface Brain and the strong emotions of the Deep Brain are important. You need a system that alerts you to problems and a system that interprets the warning and solves the issues. Awareness helps you understand what your Deep Brain is alerting to. Because emotions are experienced initially as strong physical sensations, the exploratory phase of Awareness begins by focusing on the physical component of strong emotions, as Dr. Gottman discovered in his Love Lab.

The Love Lab

John Gottman is one of the world's most influential relationship researchers. If you want to experience a more enriched relationship with your partner, you may want to read and study his book, *The Seven Principles for Making Marriage Work*. Dr. Gottman's laboratory is not like any research laboratory you would imagine. It is an apartment specially equipped with cameras and microphones. Gottman refers to it as his "Love Lab." As with Clayton Christensen and the Jobs To Be Done Theory, Gottman believes you learn more about people's health, in this case the health of a couple, by watching their interactions than you do by interviewing or surveying them.

Gottman and his team ask couples to spend the night in the Love Lab while being videotaped in order to help them resolve ongoing disagreements. Gottman says that fights are not the reason couples get divorced. People get divorced because of the way they fight. After decades of research, Gottman claims he can accurately predict which couples will get divorced 91 percent of the time.

One of the key elements Gottman looks for is if and how people calm themselves when they become emotionally flooded. "Emotionally flooded" is the term psychologists use to describe the psychological reaction that arises when we become overwhelmed by strong difficult emotions. In this heightened state, strong emotions overcome our ability to think clearly and rationally. We overidentify with the strong emotion and interpret the event through it alone. In the case of severe anger or anxiety, our heart rate and blood pressure increase, which often corresponds to a flushed sensation, headache and pressure in the chest.

Gottman observed that these bodily responses to difficult emotions are telling. If a spouse's heart rate increases above 100—or above eighty in athletes—they'd better watch out. In this state, people do and say the most hurtful and derogatory things. Gottman discovered that if at this point couples took a thirty-minute break to calm themselves and disengage from the strong emotion, they were able to respond in more loving and conciliatory ways.

This heightened negative emotional state and its often correspond-ing negative relational consequences are the things we want to avoid. This is why we suppress or numb difficult emotions.

While not calling it Awareness, Gottman discovered that calming the body reintroduced a more relaxed and curious way of thinking. Remember, when difficult emotions feel dangerous, scary, over-whelming or threatening, our automatic response is to resist them. Calming the body is a good way to help dampen this automatic urge. Thus, calming the body becomes the first step in Awareness.

Emotions in the Body

Other researchers have documented that strong difficult emotions consist of both mental and physical components. In 1941, Dr. Abram Kardiner described in his book, *The Traumatic Neurosis of War,* the mental state of "shellshocked" soldiers returning from the trenches of WWI. His book is considered to be the seminal work on PTSD. In his view, "The nucleus of the neurosis (PTSD) is a physioneurosis."[17] In other words, their emotional turmoil was not all in their heads. It was a mind-body phenomenon.

Dr. Bessel Van Der Kolk explains in his book, *The Body Keeps the Score,* "As long as we register emotions primarily in our heads, we can remain pretty much in control, but feelings as if our chest is caving in or we've been punched in the gut is unbearable. We'll do anything to make these awful visceral sensations go away, whether it is clinging desperately to another human being, rendering ourselves insensible with drugs or alcohol, or taking a knife to the skin to replace over-whelming emotions with definable sensations."[18] In Dr. Bessel's view, this physical component of strong emotions, the uncomfortable body

---

17   Abram Karniner. *The Traumatic Neurosis of War.* Martino Fine Books. 2012.

18   Bessel Van Der Kolk. *The Body Keeps the Score.* Penguin Books. 2014.

sensations, are part of what drive us to unhealthy coping behaviors. We want to avoid those uncomfortable sensations at all costs.

In 1988 Fritz Strack and colleagues performed an ingenious experiment using pencils. They asked subjects to hold a pencil in their mouth in one of two ways to see if it affected their mood. The first group held the end of the pencil in their mouth, causing their lips to pucker, similar to a frown. The other group was told to grasp the middle of the pencil horizontally with their teeth. The resulting facial position was similar to a smile. The researchers scored the participants' moods prior to grasping the pencil and afterwards. The group asked to hold the pencil by the tip, thus puckering, noted a decline in their mood. The group holding the pencil horizontally noted a rise in their mood. Similarly, studies show that sitting in a slumped position worsens your mood and degrades your sense of self-worth. When speakers stand erect, hold their chin high and use expansive arm gestures, they boost their confidence. The encouraging lesson is that even changing simple body positions can alter the way you experience emotions.

If the body experiences emotional trauma and adversity as well as the brain, and is a major driving force that causes us to seek relief through unhealthy behaviors, can changing the body alter how we experience emotions enough that we feel safe that they will not overtake us?

Physiology of Strong Emotions

To help understand why difficult emotions can lead you astray, it can be helpful to know how your brain processes tough situations. When you experience adversity, your sensory organs collect information from your environment. Sight, sound, taste, and touch are all processed in the thalamus. The thalamus is a structure within the brain that acts like an author, arranging individual events into a chronological storyline with a defined beginning, middle and end.

That storyline is quickly sent to the adjacent amygdala, which triggers a Fear Response Singal, like an inner fire alarm that warns you danger is imminent. Almost simultaneously, the information is processed by the hippocampus which stores memories in your internal hard drive. It is here that your brain compares your current circumstance with previous situations to see if you have any relevant memories that could help solve the problem. The Fear Signal is then sent to your body through the vagus nerve. The vagus nerve innervates your pharynx, larynx, heart, lungs, esophagus, stomach, intestinal tract, and other body parts. (Figure 3.3)

You now begin to feel what is happening to you as the sensory information in your body begins to loop back to your brain, but you still don't understand what is happening because your conscious Surface Brain is still in the dark. Several hundredths of a second after the amygdala first receives the original sensory signals, your medial prefrontal cortex (MPFC)/Surface Brain is finally included in the story. Think of your MPFC as a fire tower in search of new emerging fires. Once it detects a fire, it sends help to solve the problem. It is only now that you begin to understand what is happening, devise a plan, enact the plan, and attenuate the amygdala's fear response. Your MPFC is always the last to know.

If your body is the first to know and only later informs your Surface Brain, it makes sense that the first step in altering what you think about a situation should involve changing the signals that your body sends back to your MPFC. Calm your body, and you calm your mind.

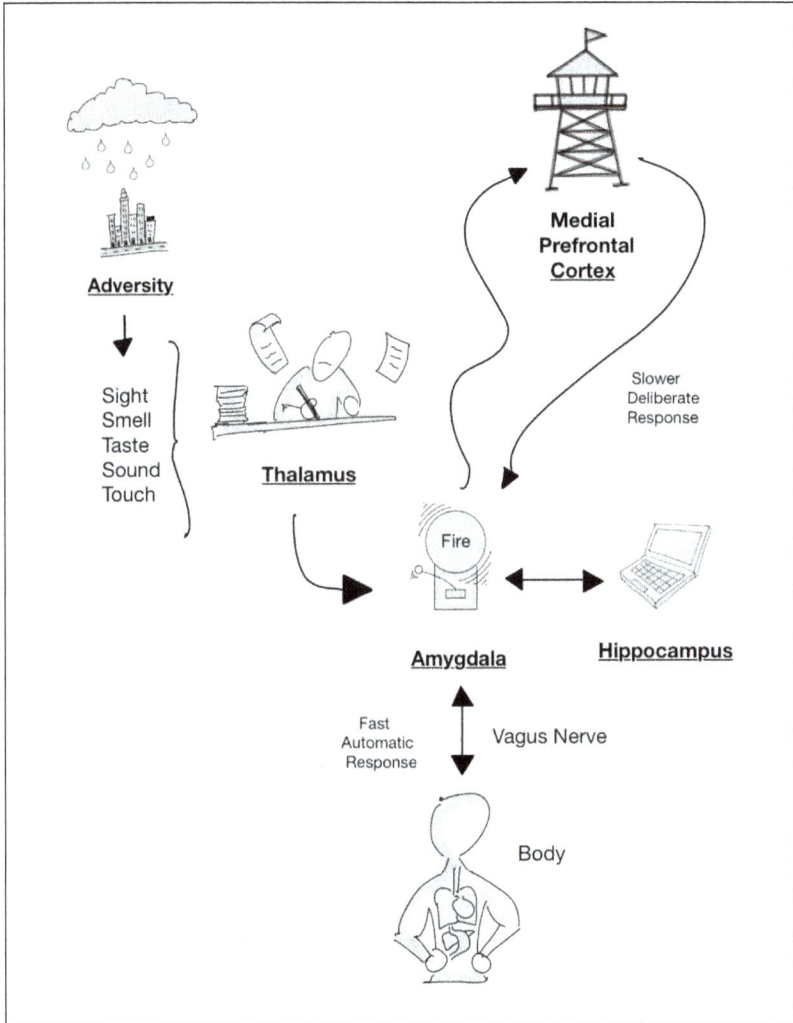

(FIGURE 3.3)

As it turns out, the vagus nerve houses two different systems, the sympathetic system and the parasympathetic system. The sympathetic system is the excitatory system. It prepares you to fight or flee. It dilates your pupils, increases your respiratory rate, increases your heart rate and the contractility of your heart, dilates the arteries that feed your skeletal muscles, activates your sweat glands, and increases your blood pressure. Part of the sympathetic system's action is the result of direct stimulation via the vagus nerve fibers and part is through activation of stress hormones like epinephrine, norepinephrine and cortisol.

The parasympathetic system has the opposite response. It is the calming system. It constricts pupils, stimulates salivation, constricts airways, decreases your heart rate and contractility, stimulates digestion, and reduces adrenal gland production of stress hormones.

With emotional flooding, as Gottman noted with his quarreling couples, the sympathetic system becomes charged by adversity. As this automatically takes control, your ability to embrace the difficult emotion and think rationally declines. The cure begins by activating your parasympathetic system, but if this is part of the automatic Deep Brain, how do you hack into it?

In the next sections, I have described four different practical but interconnected ways of hacking into your Deep Brain. The first two are fairly straightforward and easier to understand. They may be all you need. The latter two are more complex and, therefore, will take some time to understand, apply and master. The fourth technique especially is effortful to process and apply, but it is also the most powerful and introspective model.

If, after reading through the four, you find that one or two work best for you, use those and forget the others. You may even discover that by combining certain aspects of each, you will develop your own unique process. There is no right or perfect way of hacking into the Deep Brain. Use whatever method works best for you.

Awareness Hacks for the Deep Brain:

1. Three Ds

2. Mountain Observer

3. Compassionate Meditation

4. Deep Character Exploration

1. Three Ds

We've already discussed these preparatory steps in the story of Gottman's Love Lab. The three Ds provide you with a memory aid to easily recall Gottman's recommendations: Discontinue, Distance and Distract.

Let's revisit our quarreling couple. When Gottman's team sees a spouse's heart rate rise about 100, they know emotions are about to escalate. At this point, Gottman encourages couples to stop their discussion **(Discontinue),** separate into different rooms **(Distance)** and engage in activities that alter their focus **(Distract.)**

Distraction can take many forms. It can simply mean refocusing your mental attention on something different; however, I find that actually doing something different is more effective. Consider reading a book or magazine, working on a puzzle, listening to calming music, watching an enjoyable program or going for a walk. Exercise has the additional benefit of releasing your calming endorphin hormones. In Appendix II you will find a list of 365 positive activities that you can do to distract yourself. Pick one or more of the 365 or use the list to foster your own creative ideas.

After about 20-30 minutes of distancing and distraction, the sympathetic system will have calmed and you can return to work through your problems. With repetition and investment in these steps and the next techniques, you can learn to shorten the calming phase to just a few seconds.

Remember, Discontinuing/Distancing/Distracting are only preparatory steps. They help dampen difficult emotions enough that you then can process them in safe and productive ways.

2. Mountaintop Observer

Humans and other animals all experience first-order or primary emotions. These are automatically triggered by people, places, things or situations. We experience them as happiness, joy, interest, love, sadness, anger, fear, and disgust. They require no spoken language, instead they are communicated through facial expressions, tone, body habitus, and reflexive body movements. One of the things that separates humans from other animals, however, is the degree to which we experience second-order emotions. Second-order emotions are triggered by emotional knowledge, or what psychologists call "emotional schemas." These are thoughts or feelings about our emotions or how we perceive, interpret, evaluate, and respond to our emotions and the emotions of others. Because we remember what it feels like to be happy, and have concluded that happiness is a good emotion, we strive to arrange our lives so we can experience more of it. On the other hand, we remember what it feels like to fear. Our emotional schemas often pass judgment on fear as something bad, therefore we anticipate situations that may induce fear and try to avoid them.

Awareness assumes a curious compassionate role by experiencing first-order emotions as a passive observer. By freely experiencing the primary emotion without judgment, it slowly passes through your life.

When you begin to experience difficult emotions that threaten to overwhelm you, the Mountaintop Observer technique is a simple tool that will help you differentiate the rational thinking part of yourself, the Surface Brain, from the primary emotions of your Deep Brain.

Begin by closing your eyes and taking a few breaths. Visualize yourself beside a clear stream in a beautiful mountain valley. Now envision your thinking, Surface Self climbing the adjacent mountains while leaving all your emotions in the valley. When you reach the top, turn back and concentrate on the stream running through the valley floor. Visualize a specific difficult emotion floating down the river as a leaf, a boat or a log. When a difficult emotion comes into sight, don't turn away; allow yourself to experience it in your body. As long as your Surface Self stays on the mountaintop, you are safe. You will not blend with the emotion. You will not become the emotion. You are the one observing the emotion. Don't let your difficult emotion pull you back down into the valley.

As your Surface Self watches your difficult emotion, remember to assume the role of a curious, compassionate observer. Watch the emotion undulate with the current. As it drifts by, pay attention to what you feel. Remember that your emotions are your Deep Brain's way of assigning value to people, places, things, and situations. They serve as messengers, and as such all emotions are good and helpful. Their role is to inform you and keep you safe.

People don't like difficult emotions, so they often resist them. We try to suppress them, numb them, or as one person told me, "I want to shoot them out of the water." Don't kill the messengers, however. If you process them for what they are—helpful messengers without judgment—listen to them and hear what they are trying to communicate to you, difficult emotions will continue to float down the river and fade in the distance. You will have embraced full Awareness. When your difficult emotions feel heard and understood, they naturally appear and disappear in this transient way.

When we resist, we get stuck. The emotion freezes in place because it feels as if you are ignoring it. It needs to know that you understand its important message. It will continue to escalate its efforts until you finally acknowledge it, validate it, feel it, and listen to it. Once you do, it will drift off and fade into the distance.

The Mountaintop Observer will keep you from feeling overwhelmed by your difficult emotions and keep your Surface-observing self from blending or overidentifying with them. Awareness in this way differentiates your Surface Self, the one experiencing the emotion, from the emotion itself. It is a single tool, however, in a much more comprehensive toolbox for successful empowered living. It is not meant to be used alone. Implement it. Use it, but continue to acquire more tools.

Many teach that living in the present moment with a mindful curious attitude is the sole path to finding contentment and happiness. They isolate themselves in mountaintop monasteries while ignoring the essence of who we are, relationship-based prospective creatures. We not only live in the moment, but are able to learn from the past and plan for the future. In fact, the human species is naturally drawn to the future. Hope resides in our ability to plan for and imagine a better tomorrow. We are created for something greater than simply isolating ourselves from the world and becoming aware. We are called to use our awareness to make the world and the lives of those around us better.

This empowered, prospective view engages the Surface Brain as an active leader, assertively guiding your behavior and thoughts. Your Surface Brain not only helps you interpret and safely feel difficult emotions, but also helps you learn from them, act on these lessons and shape positive strategies for moving forward. With this more prospective view, you engage the world and bless it with your unique gifts and your meaningful work.

3. Compassionate Meditation

The Mountaintop Observer technique works only if you feel safe enough to experience difficult emotions. Those emotions, however, may feel too strong to bear. If you have spent your life burying, numbing or suppressing, they may be so deeply submerged beneath protective layers that you subconsciously can't allow them to come to the surface. If you are in this situation, retraining your brain to safely feel and interpret what your body is communicating can help you move forward. Compassionate Meditation is another method to calm your body's response so that strong emotions feel more manageable.

Compassion is often misunderstood as a weak virtue, most often defined by its softer qualities—encouraging, soothing and acknowledging. Kristin Neff says, "Because compassion for others is a part of nurturing, especially caring for children, we may instinctively link it to more traditional feminine gender role norms."[19] To assume that compassion is weak because of these softer qualities, however, is to make a grave mistake. Compassion is a double-sided virtue. One side is defined by its softer aspects, but the other side embodies the more assertive qualities of protection, providing and motivating. Mastering both sides of compassion produces healthy self-leadership.

Multiple studies show that self-compassionate people are happier, less depressed, less anxious, more satisfied with life, more resilient in the face of adversity, stronger physically, and have healthier relationships. To many, compassion implies self-pity, weakness, selfishness, self-indulgence, and laziness. In reality, compassion builds perspective, resiliency, selflessness, and motivation.

Today, most of the real threats we face are not from external challenges. Instead, they are inner threats to our self-image and self-concept. According to Christopher Germer, these threats come in the form of harsh self-criticism. "When we feel inadequate, our self-concept becomes threatened, so we attack the problem … ourselves."[20]

When I was a child, my father raised bees. I loved the taste of fresh honey on Mom's homemade biscuits, and those are still two of my go-to comfort foods. While I like honey, I wasn't too keen on the process of robbing the bees. Something about the possibility of getting

---

19 Kristen Neff and Christopher Germer, *The Mindful Self-Compassion Workbook* (The Guilford Press, 2018).

20 Christopher Germer, *The Mindful Path to Self-Compassion: Freeing yourself from destructive thoughts and emotions* (The Guilford Press, 2009).

stung wasn't too attractive to my 12-year-old self. Come to think of it, I'm still not too fond of stinging insects. Dad didn't like getting stung either, so he meticulously gowned himself with his sting-proof suit—hat, face net, thick long-sleeve jacket, pants, and gloves.

Beekeepers compassionately protect themselves from stings, and most of us consider that reasonable. Yet, we don't always compassionately protect ourselves from the stinging effects of our difficult emotions. Bees aren't bad because they sometimes sting, and neither are your difficult emotions. In fact, both play an essential role in promoting the health of our ecosystems—bees our external ecosystem, and difficult emotions our inner ecosystem. While both are inherently good, they both require donning ourselves with protective equipment so we can enjoy the full experience.

a. Body Positioning

To begin, either sit upright in a chair, on the floor with your legs crossed, or lie flat with your legs and arms extended. The goal is to achieve an open, relaxed, neutral body position. Remember that the way you hold your body can shape the way you experience your emotions.

b. Deep Breathing

Close your eyes and slowly breathe. I find the "square" breathing technique most useful. Slowly inhale as deeply as you can for 3-4 seconds, hold it for two seconds, exhale for 3-4 seconds, hold it for two seconds, then repeat. As you slowly and intentionally breath you actively engage the parasympathetic nervous system. Pay attention to your body. Feel the air as it enters your nose and expands your lungs. Experience the release of tension as your chest collapses with exhalation. Focus on the natural undulating rhythmic sway of your body as you breathe in and breathe out.

c. Ground Yourself

Traumatic events cause some people's memory storage systems to short-circuit. Remember that the thalamus acts like an author who arranges all sensory inputs into a neat storyline with a defined beginning, middle and end. In susceptible individuals, this process breaks down. Snippets of sensory data are stored as random information. With no way to place this information in context or chronological order, the brain relives the snippet as if it were being experienced in the present tense.

Think of a war veteran who witnessed their friend being shot. The sounds, smells, sights, tastes, and other sensations of fear become jumbled in his memory. Years later while walking down a street, he hears a car backfire that sounds similar to a rifle blast. He immediately feels his heart race and a sense of overwhelming terror, exactly like the day his friend died. He relives those emotional and physical sensations, but without the rest of the context. Because his memory is devoid of the normal contextual storyline—beginning, middle and end—he experiences the war as if it were happening right then. An ordinary day in an instant becomes a terrifying moment of tragedy. That is the life of someone living with PTSD.

When allowing yourself to feel difficult emotions, start with milder sensations. Don't attempt to tackle severely intense emotions that are prone to triggering flashbacks. To help prevent this, shift your attention to the pressure points in your buttocks, back and soles of your feet. Note where your body is firmly grounded. These pressure senses remind you that you are in the present and not the past. If severely intense memories intrude into your thoughts and attempt to hijack you to the past, purposefully refocus your attention to the grounding sensations. They are your lifeline to the present moment.

(I encourage you to seek the help of a good psychologist or counselor to help you work through this process if you have a history or severe traumatic stress.)

d. Visualize

Before starting, make sure your body is calm. To help me do this, I dim the lights. If you don't have a dimmer on your main lights, turn them off and turn on a small side lamp. I sit upright on a cushioned pad, close my eyes and begin square breathing. Certain smells like vanilla and cinnamon have a calming effect for me, so I may burn a scented candle. Others like to burn incense. I like my room to be absolutely quiet, but you may like to play soothing music or recordings of blowing wind or babbling mountain streams. Do whatever works for you.

On some particularly stressful days, this is where my Compassionate Meditation begins and ends. You may be the same way—and that's okay. Part of Compassionate Meditation is learning to respect your current limits while simultaneously providing yourself with the compassion you need in the moment.

Skip visualization and proceed to Step E, Body Scan, if you are currently emotionally flooded. Visualizing details of traumatic experiences will likely accentuate these emotions. Locating difficult emotions in your body and calming them first can be helpful.

If you feel safe and comfortable to proceed, then do so. Once you are in a calm body position, firmly grounded and centered on your breathing, pick a situation that you are having difficulty processing. As I recommended with grounding, begin with a mild or moderately painful event so you can safely build your skills. Close your eyes. Visualize the storyline of a situation or a conflict that caused you stress or pain. Start at the beginning and visualize the story through to its end. Maybe it's a relationship problem, an issue at work or a financial crisis. Can you see it clearly? In Compassionate Meditation, visualization is more than merely repeating the words, pictures and thoughts of the story in your mind. It's a rich, detailed, multisensory experience that you feel in your entire body. What do you see, hear, smell, taste, and feel? Slow your thoughts down and concentrate on these physical sensations. Don't exaggerate them; experience them as if they were naturally occurring.

Note the difference in what I am asking you to do, as opposed to what people experience with PTSD. I want you to visualize the experience in its entirety, in chronological order—beginning, middle and end—not as isolated segments. The ending is especially important, because it reminds you that these adverse events were in the past. As with grounding, I encourage you to seek the help of a good psychologist or counselor if you have a history of severe traumatic stress.

Visualization can help process two types of circumstances:

1. You intermittently relive the strong emotions of a past adverse event.

2. You want to practice relaxation skills for what you anticipate to be a stressful situation in the future.

e. Body Scan

Now that you are beginning to embrace difficult emotions, it's time to locate them, identify them and name them. Assume the mindset of an investigative reporter. Become curious about your emotions, but don't let yourself be so overwhelmed and consumed by them that you can't keep an objective perspective. I like to use the Mountaintop Observer mediation before doing my body scan to help keep my observing self differentiated from my difficult emotions.

Close your eyes, calm your breathing and curiously search your body for emotional sensations. Where do you feel them? Can you isolate them and describe them or name them? If so, great—keep a mental log of these sensations so you can quickly identify them in the future.

If you are new to this, you may feel a little lost or overwhelmed. If you have a history of chronically suppressing and numbing difficult feelings, you especially may benefit from a more systematic approach. A therapist friend of mine, Theresa Moore, introduced me to the Body Scan. This helps you safely and non-judgmentally reconnect with your physical self while not overlooking any subtle sensations.

Start with your toes and feet. Do you feel anything uncomfortable there? If so, can you describe it? Does it tingle, burn, stab, cramp or buzz? Do you feel heat, cold, pressure or tightness? Maybe that part of your body merely feels hollow. Describe it in your own words. Take your time. This is not a race. Once you have experienced all there is to feel, contract your toes and feet tightly for several seconds then relax. Note the contrast between how your body feels as the tension builds and then as it releases once you relax.

As you relax your body, you calm your mind. Next, move up to your calves and do the same. Continue the same process until you finish at the top of your head. Make a list of all the uncomfortable sensations you identified and any difficult emotions you associated with them. If you can't associate any difficult emotions, don't worry about it. This is a learning process. For now, simply list your uncomfortable body sensations and where you felt them.

For some of you, reconnecting with your body may feel frightening or unsafe. If you feel like you are beginning to feel overwhelmed, return to your grounding points. Concentrate on the sensations in your bottom, back and feet. Those pressure points and their corresponding sensations are your anchors to the present.

Return to your breathing and the sensations of air entering your lungs and the release as they collapse. Return to the rhythmic sway of your body as you breathe in and breathe out. If you feel secure, return to the body part that was giving you trouble, or move on to another area. If you still feel unsafe or overwhelmed, I encourage you to stop and secure the help of a counselor. They can help you navigate these tumultuous experiences safely.

If you don't feel like you need a counselor, but want more details of how to assume a curious, self-compassionate mindset, Kristin Neff's *The Mindful Self-Compassion Workbook* is one of my favorite resources.

f. Acknowledge

Now you have identified a few strong emotions and allowed yourself to feel their corresponding body components, it is important to heal these with compassionate words. This next step requires you to validate what you feel. Acknowledgment allows you to turn toward the pain, recognize it for what it is—a moment of suffering—and heal it.

Most of us find it much easier to brush the pain aside and move on. It's part of our western culture. We've been told all our lives to suck it up and pull ourselves up by our bootstraps. Movie heroes frequently yell back to their foe or the universe, "Is that all you got?" In reality, we rarely want more pain than is already being thrown at us, and we certainly don't feel the need to antagonize it.

The childhood saying, "Sticks and stones may break my bones, but words will never hurt me," sounds good when spoken, but deep inside we understand it's a lie. Words do matter. Words carry just as many consequences as behaviors.

Trauma and adversity is never felt more acutely and widespread as in times of war. Winston Churchill was a brilliant war strategist, a dedicated student of history and, most importantly, a master of the power of language. Much of the reason that the allies won WWII was because of Churchill's efforts to help sustain the British people's morale, especially during the height of German bombing in 1940. When he spoke about the war, he spoke honestly. He didn't minimize the British people's suffering. He acknowledged the hardships they had endured and would continue to face, as well as the sacrifices they would be forced to make.

In 1932, Churchill told the House of Commons, "Tell the truth to the British people. They are a tough people, a robust people. They may be a bit offended at the moment, but if you have told them exactly what is going on, you have insured yourself against the complaints and the reproaches, which are very unpleasant when they come home on the morrow of some disillusionment."[21]

Churchill's acknowledgment of Britain's precarious situation and its people's suffering mattered and so does your acknowledgment of your own suffering. Always be honest with yourself. Don't be tempted to ignore the harsh truth or soften it with lies. Your deep self knows the truth anyway. Admit that times are tough and that there will be more tough times to come. Validate your pain.

Kristin Neff recommends that you say something to yourself like:

- "This hurts."

- "This is painful."

- "This is stressful."

- "This is a moment of suffering."

Maybe that sounds too fluffy or soft for you. If so, envision yourself receiving a personal radio address from Churchill at the height of your adversity. What would Churchill suggest that you acknowledge to yourself? Maybe something like this:

- "I am experiencing a cruel, heart-rending struggle."

- "I have nothing to offer myself but blood, toil, tears, and sweat. I have before me an ordeal of the most grievous kind."

---

21 Winston Churchill, Speech to the House of Commons, 1932.

- "Like my forefathers before me, who fought against the tyranny of Hitler's fascism, and Stalin's communism, I stand at the perilous, perplexing, precipice of history, facing the undaunted foes of darkness."

Maybe that's a little over the top. The point is to find language that feels right to you. What words do you need to hear?

g. *Common Humanity*

Each of us is part of humanity's communal suffering, and each of us is part of the collective solution. Each of us is worthy and plays an integral part in alleviating each other's suffering. This can only happen when we intentionally stay connected to others. When we remove ourselves from the common experience, we isolate ourselves and salvation becomes a selfish endeavor.

Several recent studies suggest a disturbing trend. Younger generations are becoming depressed at a much higher rate than older ones. Martin Seligman, previous president of the American College of Psychology and author of *Learned Optimism*, believes that much of this is the result of two related issues: "Elevation of the Self" and "Loss of the Commons."

> "The life committed to nothing larger than itself is a meager life. Human beings require a context of meaning and hope. We used to have ample context, and when we encountered failure, we could pause and take our rest in that setting and revive our sense of who we are. I call that larger setting the commons. It consists of a belief in the nation, in God, in one's family, or in a purpose that transcends our lives."[22]

---

22   Martin Seligman, *Learned Optimism: How to Change Your Mind and Your Life* (Vintage, Reprint edition, 2006).

For the last few decades, many mental health experts have taught that improving the self-esteem of young people, elevation of the self, produces healthy, successful and well-adjusted adults. Unfortunately, this advice has been a disaster. Self-esteem is a conditional feeling of self-worth based on a comparison to others. It promotes the selfish idea that in order for you to succeed, others must lose.

Not only does self-esteem promote selfish behavior, but it also promotes an unstable foundation for mental health based on conditional factors. What happens when you inevitably fail to excel? What happens when your performance drops below average? Nobody can be above average in everything all the time. There will always be other people who are prettier, stronger, faster, more wealthy, and more popular than you.

Because a comparison scarcity mentality robs people of rich relationships and adequate self-caring techniques, people turn to artificial means of boosting self-esteem through unkind acts of prejudice or of self-gratification. Prejudice artificially elevates our social group, gender, race or economic group above others to falsely make ourselves feel special. Prejudice not only hurts the people you demean, but it also hurts you by distancing you from the commonality of the human experience.

Self-gratification is self-esteem's right-hand assistant. As self-esteem shifts the responsibility from an internal process of self-care to a focus on exterior factors, it becomes the responsibility of others and external things to make you happy. In a day and age of consumerism, marketers relentlessly sell us on the idea that a product or service exists to meet every need. When self-esteem fails and we feel less than worthy, it's easy to look to material things to solve our problems. External things may temporarily help, but we quickly adapt to their mood-elevating effects. Remember the homeostasis of dopamine.

Another problem with the self-esteem movement is that as people become more self-absorbed, they stop investing in things bigger than themselves. They stop investing in the basic institutions that link us with other people, such as family, faith and the nation. With loss of connection, intense adversities heighten feelings of isolation. Subsequently, you may feel that these burdens are yours alone to carry. A vicious, dark cycle ensues. You not only become lost in your own pain, but you also become blind to the struggles of others, even further isolating yourself.

Empowered self-care acknowledges that we are all united in a similar common struggle. No matter your race, gender, socioeconomic level or religion, we all suffer. None of us is so special that we exit life without experiencing pain. In this way we are all connected.

Unlike many modern political leaders who promote division through identity politics, another reason Winston Churchill is celebrated as one of history's greatest leaders is because of his ability to unite the British people and the allies toward a common purpose. His words, while sometimes graphic, clearly note that he was personally dedicated to fighting with the British people:

> "If this long island story of **ours** is to end at last, let it end only when **each one of us** lies choking in his own blood upon the ground."

> "Even though large tracts of Europe and many old and famous States have fallen or may fall into the grip of the Gestapo and all the odious apparatus of Nazi rule, **we** shall not flag or fail. **We** shall go on to the end. **We** shall fight in France, we shall fight on the seas and oceans, **we** shall fight with growing confidence and growing strength in the air, **we** shall defend our island, whatever the cost may be. **We** shall fight on the beaches, **we** shall fight on the landing grounds, **we** shall fight in the fields and in the streets, **we** shall fight in the hills; **we** shall never surrender."[23]

23 Winston Churchill, Speech to the House of Commons June 4, 1940.

The struggle was to be endured and fought together. They were not alone, and the only solution depended on their collective efforts.

We too live a common struggle. **We** all experience adversity. **We** all feel pain. The natural dysfunctional tendency is to blame our problems on external causes, our environments, our situations or what other people do. Sometimes external circumstances do need to change, as in the case of physical and emotional abuse, but your external world changes most effectively when you assume the healthy mindset of changing yourself first.

Common Humanity in meditation has two arms:

1. Remind yourself that you are not alone. You are not the first or only person to experience suffering. Repeat these phrases or develop similar phrases that resonate better with your situation:

    "Suffering is a part of life."
    "Everyone experiences similar feelings."
    "I'm not alone."
    "Nobody is exempt from suffering, including me."

2. Focus outside yourself. To enhance your connection with the rest of humanity, intentionally scale down your innate importance. List a few meaningful things you can do for others. What can you intentionally sacrifice for the good of the commons? As you meditate, picture yourself doing these things.

h. Soothing Touch

A psychiatrist friend of mine who frequently counsels couples commonly prescribes what she calls "skin therapy." She encourages couples, in the privacy of their own home, to frequently embrace each other free of clothing's impediments. As you can understand, this often leads to even more intimate physical connection. Even without sexual connection, the touch of bare skin strengthens couples' emotional connections.

Skin therapy, albeit a different form, is used in obstetrical suites as well. Immediately after delivery, nurses place babies in the warm embrace of their mother's breasts. Skin-to-skin contact stimulates the release of oxytocin, which promotes bonding between individuals.

Even in much less exposed ways, physical touch can promote healing. In my Internal Medical practice, I employ the healing power of appropriate touch regularly through the simple act of examining a patient. By placing my hands on a person, I communicate that they are important. Have you ever been to a cold, sterile doctor's office where the physician sat on the opposite side of the room and never touched you? How healing did that feel? Contrast that to the last time you felt down and somebody you love gave you a big hug.

Today we understand the innate need for loving touch, but it hasn't always been that way. Prior to the mid-1950s, psychologists believed that babies were drawn to their mothers solely for nourishment and that too much affection could be harmful to children. Love and social and intellectual development were believed to be separate entities that did not influence each other. The predominant wisdom of the time was that your intelligence and personality were entirely encoded in your genes. The theory held that the most important thing children needed was a clean, sterile, structured environment for their natural intelligence and personality to blossom. Affection, encouragement and guidance only inhibited the child's ability to discover the best path for themselves. Orphanages during this era were intentionally designed devoid of nurturing tendencies lest they spoil the child. It was a disaster.

Most of what we understand about human affection and physical touch stands in stark contrast to those early beliefs because of the work of Harry Harlow. Harlow had been studying the behaviors of macaque monkeys for years, but the process of acquiring the monkeys was expensive and when they arrived, they were often malnourished and diseased. Once in his lab, their diseases quickly spread to their new cage mates and playmates.

Following the best theory of child development at the time, Harlow separated the monkeys into individual cages to prevent the spread of disease. Even young babies were separated from their mothers. The cages were kept fastidiously clean and sterile. Because Harlow and his team separated the babies from their mothers, they were forced to develop an artificial formula and ways of feeding them.

To explore an idea he had about why monkeys often failed to thrive in captivity, Harlow built two types of surrogate mothers for his isolated baby monkeys. One was constructed of bare wire metal and the other was made of soft cloth. In each cage, he placed both surrogate monkeys, but an artificial feeding tube only ran through the metal wire mother. The soft cloth mother sat in the opposite corner and provided nothing more than something with which to cuddle.

Paradoxical to the current wisdom, the baby monkeys overwhelmingly preferred the cloth surrogate mother. The only time they approached the wire mother was to feed. Even then, many of the babies tightly clinched the soft cloth mother while stretching across the cage to reach the feeding tube.

Physical contact was a need that they desperately attempted to maintain, despite the difficulty and discomfort of doing so. Unfortunately, as these isolated monkeys aged, it became apparent that the need for reciprocal touch, something an inanimate cloth surrogate could not provide, was also required. Many of his ill-raised lonely babies became psychotic, dysfunctional and depressed adults.

Harlow made two important discoveries with this single series of experiments. Primates not only need to feel something soft and warm, but—just as importantly—they need reciprocal touch in return.

Soothing touch even in the absence of someone who can give you a hug is not without merit. Self-soothing touch is a technique you can use to calm yourself during your personal meditation time. When you calm yourself, you think more rationally. When you think more rationally, you engage in more socially acceptable behavior that encourages others to reach out to you.

Self-soothing touch sounded a little too weird for me the first time I read about it. I was skeptical and, honestly, felt a little stupid even thinking about it. Eventually I decided it was worth a try, but made sure I was by myself so nobody could see me. I experience anxiety in my chest. It feels like an expanding balloon that is about to explode. I thought, "What do I have to lose?" I sat up straight, took several deep breaths, grounded my body to the floor, allowed myself to feel the discomfort, and placed my right hand on the center of my chest. I almost immediately felt a sense of calm and was surprised at how impactful it was.

Neff has experimented with many different forms of touch and has discovered that no one technique works for everybody. She suggests you experiment until you discover what specific technique comforts you and makes you feel safe.

Below are some of her suggestions:

- One hand over your heart

- Two hands over your heart

- Gently stroking your chest

- Cupping your hand over a fist over your heart

- One hand on your heart and one on your belly

- Two hands on your belly

- One hand on your cheek

- Gently stroking your arms

- Crossing your arms and giving yourself a gentle hug

- One hand tenderly holding the other

- Cupping your hands in your lap

While compassionate meditation can be used during a specific traditional meditative session, it can be thought of more broadly as a continuous way of being, a way of engaging your normal daily life, including the way you commune with others. In this way, a simple handshake or hug extends the more expansive definition of meditation to common ways of bonding with others.

As the COVID pandemic of 2019 spread, we became fearful of touching and meeting with each other. Our most vulnerable populations, those in nursing homes, were among those hit the hardest. Individuals already isolated from their families and society became even more secluded and, unsurprisingly, the rates of depression soared. In our attempts to protect them, like the orphans of the 1930s and 1940s, the cure created its own menacing monster. Some lessons we learn slowly.

While you can't force others to spontaneously embrace you, you can initiate the process. You can, more importantly, become the type of person that people want to embrace. By becoming more loving, you create a positive feedback loop that fosters further engagement and healing. None of us is meant to live in isolation.

Sometimes communion and connection with other people is not as available or possible as you may like or need. Pet therapy is another great way to experience the healing power of touch. Like humans, animals have the additional benefit of providing reciprocal touch. Dogs especially make good therapy pets because they naturally crave attention from members of their "pack."

Remember, however, that the goal of self-soothing touch, and even pet therapy, is not merely to dampen your difficult emotions. The goal of these tools is to help you establish and maintain a healthy relationship with your own thoughts and emotions in order to estab-lish and maintain healthy relationships with others.

i. Encouraging and Comforting words

As you embrace strong emotions during compassionate meditation, another tool you can use to keep them from overwhelming you is to employ encouraging and comforting words. In moments of crisis, we all need to feel understood. We wish somebody could listen to us and bathe us with kind, soothing words. We need to hear that we are loved, that we are worthy, that our lives matter. Unfortunately, we don't always have somebody to tell us these things in the moment. This is where you can take leadership of your own needs and tell yourself the things you need to hear.

In our western culture we emphasize treating others with kind-ness, dignity and respect. Central to that is the golden rule, "Do unto others as you would have them do unto you."[24] Yet we forget about treating ourselves with the same kindness, dignity and respect that we offer up so generously. We tell ourselves the most hurtful, deroga-tory things that we would never utter to the people we love. When your inner critic screams at you or your cruel inner judge passes down harsh verdicts, assume the persona of a compassionate friend. What would that friend tell you? What words would they use? What tone would they adopt? Or as the golden rule encourages, what would you tell a loved one who was experiencing a similar situation? Would you use the same words, tone and posture that you use with yourself?

Self-compassion allows you to become your inner ally instead of an inner enemy. What are your emotions telling you that you need to hear? How do those inner voices reflect your basic needs of affec-tion, autonomy, freedom, inclusion, safety, creative work, identity,

---

24 Luke 6:31.

sustenance (food, water, shelter), mastery, or rest, recovery and recreation? Maybe you have denied yourself encouraging words for so long that your Deep Brain is crying out for all of these. Note that these needs are not simple individual wants or desires. They are not optional, and they are common to us all. You are not exempt.

How can you phrase these basic needs as encouraging words or mantras?

Here's my attempt:

- May I feel love and worthiness.

- May I feel free to choose my response and direction.

- May I feel included and cherished.

- May I feel safe physically and emotionally.

- May I discover and understand my unique creative purpose.

- May I live into my own identity.

- May I feel empowered to pursue mastery.

- May I understand how to meet my physical and emotional needs and the needs of others.

- May I give myself permission to rest and recover.

What do you wish a loved one would tell you? How can you frame your unmet needs as wishes or desires?

- "It's okay to slow down."

- "I don't have to perform or achieve to be accepted."

- "I am worthy."

- "I am enough."

Kirsten Neff suggests:

"May I be safe.
May I be happy.
May I be healthy.
May I live with ease."[25]

Maybe you need to hear something less soft, but more motivating and encouraging, something like Churchill would say in moments of battle:

"I will fight on the seas ...
I will fight in the air ...
I will fight on the beaches ...
I will fight on the landing grounds ...
In the end, I will prevail!"[26]

If you like these more forceful words, just make sure your fight is to embrace your difficult emotions and change yourself, instead of resisting the emotion and trying to force others and the world around you to change to your expectations.

The important thing is to use words that resonate with you and encourage you to become a better version of yourself.

Compassionate Meditation Overview

   a. Calm body position

   b. Deep breathing

   c. Grounding

25 Kristen Neff, *The Mindful Self-Compassion Workbook: A Proven Way to Accept Yourself, Build Inner Strength, and Thrive* (The Guilford Press, 2018).

26 Winston Churchill, Speech to the House of Commons, June 4, 1940.

d. Visualization

e. Body scan

f. Acknowledgement and validation

g. Common humanity

h. Soothing touch

i. Comforting words

4. Deep Character Exploration (DCE)

Researcher and professor Michael Gazzaniga used projected images to discover that the brain is divided into two connected but independent halves. In his book *The Social Brain*, Gazzaniga contends that the human brain is not simply divided into two parts, i.e. a right brain and a left brain. Instead, our brains are much more segmented into an undetermined number of independently functioning modules. Accordingly, our emotional and cognitive lives are shaped by how these independent modules relate to each other. Gazzaniga says, "Metaphorically speaking, we humans are more of a sociological entity than a unified psychological entity—we have a social brain." He goes on to explain, "The mind is not an indivisible whole operating in a single way ... These modular activities frequently operate apart from our conscious verbal selves."[27]

He views the Surface Brain as a single acting module and the Deep Brain as a confederation of independent modules. The role of the Surface Brain is to interpret and construct theories that explain the behaviors of the various independent, subconscious, non-verbal modules of the Deep Brain.

---

27 Michael Gazzaniga, *The Social Brain* (Basic Books: Discovering the Networks of the Mind, 1985)

Consistent with this theory, psychologist Dr. Richard Schwartz developed a type of psychotherapy based on his experience as a family therapist that he calls Internal Family Systems Therapy. As early as the 1980s, he began to notice that his clients described their various inner entities as parts, saying, "Part of me feels ... " When I read this it rang true to me, and I thought about when I lived in Tennessee and was thinking about moving back to Texas. I remember that part of me wanted to stay in Tennessee where I had several state and national parks to backpack, kayak and mountain bike, but another part of me was looking forward to a new job opportunity and being more centrally located between my wife's family and my family. Part of me wanted to stay and at the same time part of me wanted to go. I suspect you have had similar feelings and may have even used that exact "part of me" language too.

Each of these inner parts represents or arises from a unique area of your Deep Brain, as Gazzaniga described with his social mental modules. Much like members of a large family, each part seems to act independently, but is also connected to the other parts.

Schwartz opens his book, *Internal Family Systems Therapy*, with an anecdote from his own life. He tells the story of how he began to excitedly share his book with his father. He says, "My father looked at me from behind his newspaper and said, 'That sounds good,' in a flat, distracted tone. I felt a surge of resentment slide up from my gut, making my face flush and my head throb."[28] Notice the signs of emotional flooding that we discussed earlier. He continues, "Suddenly the affection and excitement I had been enjoying disappeared. 'He just doesn't care about my work,' I thought. 'He never cared about my ideas or about me.' I looked again at my father's face, and it seemed harder and more angular. Somewhere inside, I had a vague sense

---

28   Richard Schwartz, Internal Family Systems Therapy (The Guilford Press, 1997).

that I was overreacting, but this didn't stop me from storming out of the room, vowing to myself again to never talk to my father about the book."[29]

Schwartz asks himself, "What happened here? Did I simply lose my temper? In a sense, I changed temporarily into a very different person, complete with different feelings and thoughts, but also different ways of sensing and seeing the world and of moving and talking [...] Am I the resentful person or the affectionate one, or both? Or am I the one who knew I was overacting?"[30]

According to Gazzaniga, Schwartz was all the above. Part of him was angry, part was affectionate and part acted as the surface/outside observer looking in. Historically, the mental health system has labeled people as if they were monolithic, single entities that were defined by their most pathologic tendencies. We label people as being majorly depressed, generally anxious, bipolar, narcissistic or suffering from PTSD. We pathologize people, making them dependent on the system for healing. When people view themselves as a solitary personality and then experience difficult emotions and thoughts, they believe those extreme thoughts and feelings represent the whole of who they are.

Internal Family Systems Therapy emphasizes that while your strong difficult emotions and thoughts are a part of you, each constitutes only a small part of who you are. As a human, you experience a plethora of emotions and thoughts, including positive ones like joy, love and curiosity. No single emotion defines you. The other exciting revelation of this model is that while we all harbor constraining beliefs and thoughts, we also possess all the parts we need to heal ourselves. Sometimes we just need help releasing those resources.

---

29 Richard Schwartz, Internal Family Systems Therapy (The Guilford Press, 1997).

30 Richard Schwartz, Internal Family Systems Therapy (The Guilford Press, 1997).

When Pixar made the animated movie *Inside Out*, they did a fabulous job creating a structure for children and adults to describe and discuss their feelings, similar to Internal Family Systems Therapy. The movie is about a young girl, Riley, and her journey to cope with adversity. Riley's conscious self, or what I have referred to as your Surface Self/Surface Brain, narrates the movie as an observer looking in from the outside in asking, "Do you ever look at someone and wonder, what is going on inside their head? Well, I know. Hey, well, I know Riley's head."[31]

From the beginning, the story emphasizes the importance of curiosity and an inner emotional awareness. Riley personifies her emotions as individual characters. Brilliantly, the producers and writers mirror the concrete thinking of children as she simply names her inner characters after the primary human emotions Joy, Sadness, Anger, Disgust, and Fear. Note that of the five emotions in the movie only one is positive, Joy, mirroring the reality that difficult emotions are 3-5 times more powerful than positive ones.

As I thought about all these things—Dr. Schwartz's technique of uncovering our inner family of parts; Dr. Gazzaniga's description of the brain as a social confederation of independent modules; *Inside Out's* use of cartoon characters to represent our individual emotions; Kristin Neff's idea of compassion resembling the mindset of a curious explorer; and my own analogy of the brain floating like an iceberg with its surface portion exposed above the water and its deeper parts hidden below—I wondered if in searching for a process to safely explore our Deep Brain's hidden parts we could learn something from an actual exploration. As usual, history became one of my greatest teachers and inspirations.

---

31 Peter Docter, *Inside Out* (Pixar, 2015).

In the early hours of April 15, 1912 in the North Atlantic, one of maritime's greatest peacetime tragedies occurred. In all of their hubris, the builders portrayed this ship as unsinkable. On its maiden voyage from Southampton, England to New York, at 11:40 p.m. on April 14, the Titanic hit an iceberg, rupturing five of its 16 watertight compartments. It could have stayed afloat if no more than four compartments had flooded. With five compartments breached, however, it sank in a little over two hours, killing over 1,500 people.

For years, the location of the Titanic's grave was a mystery. I remember as a child being enthralled with the story, never thinking that in my lifetime the puzzle would be solved. In 1985, a joint American-French exploration team, led by Dr. Robert Ballard of the Massachusetts-based Woods Hole Oceanographic Institution, discovered the Titanic 370 miles south of Newfoundland in two separate pieces. Its final resting place was 13,000 feet, or 2.5 miles, below the surface.

At the time, the public didn't know the full nature of the mission. *National Geographic* was only able to reveal the full story after documents of the expedition were unclassified by the US Navy. The Titanic expedition was a small part of a top-secret Cold War mission to test a new robotic camera technology called Argo. Towed behind a surface ship, Argo was capable of descending to depths of 20,000 feet, making 98 percent of the oceans' floors accessible for the first time.

Robert Ballard had asked the US Navy to help him finance and build Argo, but the Navy was not interested in helping him hunt for the Titanic. They were interested, however, in using his technology to survey the wrecks of two nuclear submarines that had been lost in the 1960s, the USS Thresher and Scorpion. The Navy finally agreed that if he could prove his technology by locating and mapping their lost submarines, he could use whatever time remained in the expedition to search for the Titanic.

Here's an excerpt from the *National Geographic* article:

"Ballard's military project left him with just 12 days to look for Titanic, but it had also given him an idea for a new search technique. While photographing Thresher and Scorpion, he'd noticed that the current had carried small bits of wreckage from the ships as they fell to the seafloor, creating a long chain of debris. With this in mind, he decided not to search for the Titanic's hull. Instead, he would use Argo (a new underwater submersible) to scour the bottom for its much larger debris trail (parts), which might stretch as far as a mile. He found he could use it to track down the ship itself.

After several grueling days, they were rewarded with the sight of riveted hull plates and the telltale boiler. Argo continued stalking the debris trail, and the following morning, Titanic's bow came looming out of the inky depths."[32]

History's lessons can be so rich if we only pay attention. The Titanic was never going to reveal her secrets until explorers discovered new tools, technologies and techniques. Even when these technologies became possible it still took a highly motivated individual who persevered despite mounting obstacles to promote their development, learn how to use them, adapt the technologies to unique settings, and be willing to risk failure to pursue a goal.

As with Ballard's Titanic expedition, your inner journey requires similar qualities:

1. Be willing to use unconventional tools and techniques.

2. Learn how to use these new tools.

3. Adapt these tools and techniques to your specific situation.

---

32 Evan Andrews, *The Real Story Behind the Discovery of Titanic's Watery Grave* (National Geographic, April 17, 2017).

4. Allow yourself to become vulnerable and take risks.

5. Act deliberately and with perseverance.

Deep within each of us lies a society of—using the language of Dr. Richard Schwartz—diverse specialized parts, or—like *Inside Out*—inner characters. These inner parts or characters naturally want to coalesce into a unified powerful civilization, or a social confederation. Our inner civilization, when working cooperatively, capitalizes on each inner character's unique gifts and skill sets. Most peoples' inner characters, however, play polarized or dysfunctional roles which yield strife and discord.

Deep Character Exploration (DCE) is my twist on Dr. Schwartz's Internal Family Systems Therapy. It is a way of exploring your Deep Brain that helps you safely identify all your inner parts, learn how each part communicates, discover what each part needs, and helps your Surface Self meet their needs in healthier ways. Searching for your individual inner parts, similar to Ballard's search for smaller parts of the Titanic, will lead you to an amazing treasure, a unified self that works synchronously together.

With DCE, you envision your inner parts, emotions, feelings or thoughts as characters or citizens of a deep, hidden underwater civilization or society. Inner parts may assume either human or non-human forms. Sometimes they will morph from one to another as your perspective of them changes. For this reason, "characters" may be a more accurate and inclusive term than citizens. As an example, one of my inner parts—Anger—initially felt like a monster rising from deep within. As I gained better perspective, it morphed into a stern-faced sentry, establishing and guarding personal boundaries. We'll talk more about this morphing process later.

Think of this unique process of envisioning not as imagining a pretend world, but as looking through a window at a real inner world.

In it your inner parts are not fictional characters, but real aspects of your true personality, your true character. These inner parts are the independently functioning modules of your Deep Brain, to which Gazzaniga referred.

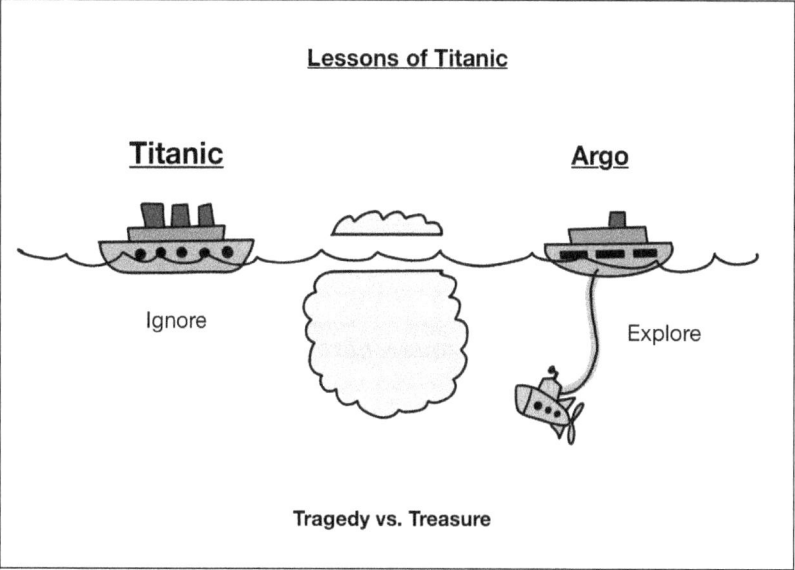

(FIGURE 3.4)

The words you use are important, so I call this special form of envisioning, "in-visioning," short for inner vision. In Deep Character Exploration, you in-vision the Surface Self as an explorer who operates a ship on the surface of a large ocean. This surface world is the world of awareness. The Deep Self is composed of an underwater society of characters who live and interact in the subaquatic world of the subconscious.

Don't feel like you must use all aspects of this tool for it to work. Use the bits that resonate with you and discard the rest. Likewise, as you use this tool, be open to your own voice of creativity and inspiration. If you discover a way of in-visioning your inner self that resonates better with you, use it.

To give you an example of what this looks like, meet my Surface Self and Deep Self:

Surface Self: *Curious Explorer*

Humans can consciously think of only one thing at a time, therefore, you experience your conscious Surface Self as a single agent. This agent's purpose is to interpret your inner characters' behavior, guide your behavior and investigate the world around you. Therefore, I visualize my conscious self as a curious world explorer. At times I will refer to this part as the Self, Surface Self, Surface Brain or simply Self.

Deep Self: *Civilization of Inner Characters*

The Deep Self is a more complex system. It subconsciously engages multiple thoughts, feelings, emotions, and sensations simultaneously. I, therefore, visualize my Deep Self as a society of inner characters:

- Thomas Edison
- Dr. Spock
- Hippy
- Sad Boy
- Happy Playful Boy
- Angry Monster
- Judge
- Mother Teresa
- Chameleon

When I am leading myself in a healthy, respectful, compassionate way, I see myself like this:

Modular Mind

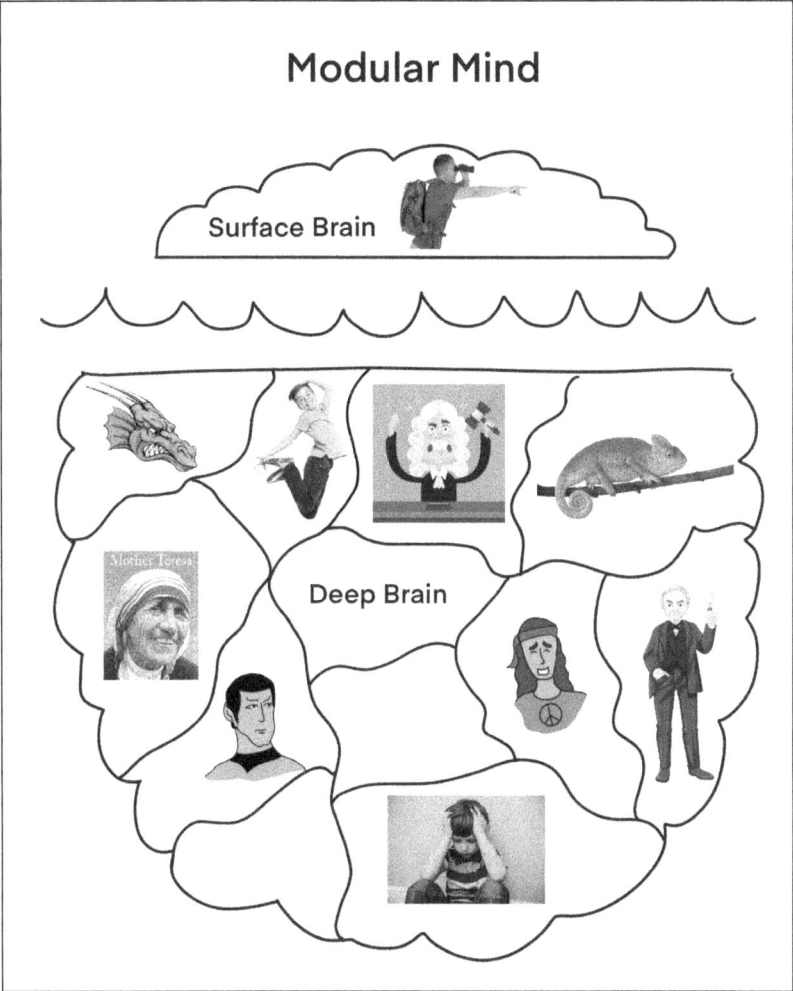

Surface Brain

Deep Brain

(FIGURE 3.5)

When I over identify or blend with a single difficult emotion, I see the world monolithically. I see myself only through the eyes of that single part of me. That looks like:

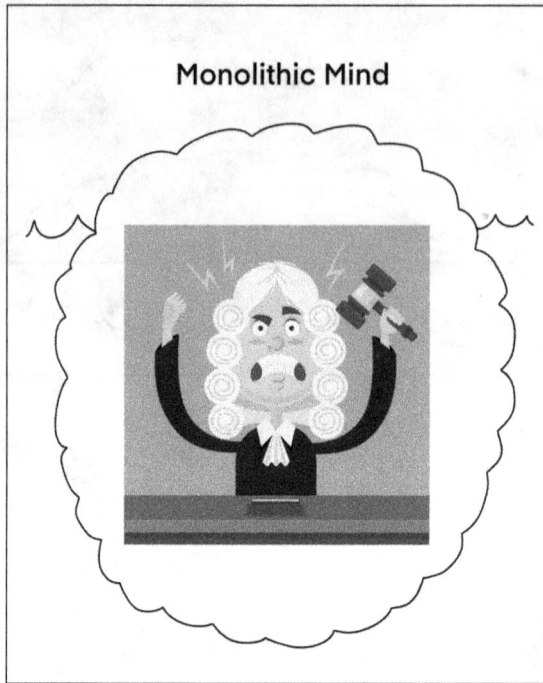

Monolithic Mind

(FIGURE 3.6)

Now it's your turn. Close your eyes, assume a calm body posture, take several deep breaths, note any sensations in your body to which you need to pay attention. If you need to provide yourself with soothing touch or comforting words, take the time to do so. When you're ready to proceed, in-vision yourself boarding a new, technologically advanced submersible. It could be a submarine, a new type of diving suit or something entirely different. If confined spaces bother you, in-vision your Surface Self sitting on the open deck of a surface ship looking at the camera monitors of your new remote submersible, like Argo.

The vehicle you select isn't important. The only thing that matters is that you feel comfortable with it. Take a moment to get to know your new submersible. How does it look, sound, feel, and smell? Explore it until you feel comfortable progressing. This new mental tool allows your Surface Self to explore your deep underworld in safety. It creates enough mental distance and separation between your Surface Self and your Deep Brain's inner parts, like the Mountaintop Observer, that it prevents blending or overidentification with your emotions, yet it still allows enough access that you can experience and get to know them.

1. Identify Your Surface Self

You may find it easiest to begin by identifying a character that represents your Surface Self. Think of your ideal observing self as a compassionate, non-judgmental, yet curious leader. What does that intentional leader look like to you? Maybe, like me, it's a famous explorer such as Robert Ballard or Jacques Cousteau. Maybe your surface leader looks more like a famous movie director, political hero, astute business leader, spiritual leader or a movie character. As always, choose the one that feels most fitting for you. Once you settle on a character, draw a picture of it or find an image in a magazine or on the internet and cut it out or print it.

2. Identify Your Deep Self's Inner Parts

Given the more complex nature of the Deep Self, this process is a bit more involved. You may even need a little help to encourage your inner parts to express themselves. Because we most often struggle with our difficult emotions and parts, you may want to begin by identifying those first. Visualize yourself dealing with a difficult situation from your past or facing a potentially difficult situation in the future. Maybe you had a fight with your spouse, or have a presentation to make in front of a large crowd next week. As we discussed before, start with a less intense issue you feel safe exploring. As you visualize this scenario, return to your body for a moment. What emotions, feelings or sensations are you experiencing? Where are they in your body?

In your mind's eye, slip your submersible into the water and slowly descend. Direct your submersible to these body sensations. As you do this, remember that your Surface Self either remains on the surface ship's deck or is protected within the steel walls of your submersible. Now move to your nearest porthole or fire up one of the cameras. Imagine that they are equipped with hi-tech sensors that help translate your feelings and emotions into visual images. Allow yourself to fully experience this emotion in your body.

Can you begin to recognize any of your inner emotions? Is anything coming into focus? What type of characters do they look like—a person, a cartoon character, an animal, a monster, a geometric shape, an artistic design or a color? If you can, try to draw a picture that represents what you feel. You don't need to be a great artist for this to work. Your pictures don't even need to look like anything in particular. Another way to translate your physical emotional sensations into images is to scour the internet or magazines for images that represent what you are feeling. When you find one, print it or cut it out. I especially like the idea of representing emotions as movie characters.

If you still can't in-vision the feeling clearly, that's okay; try to put a name to what you are feeling. You can work with it as long as you can identify in some way what you are feeling. The Feeling Wheel (Figure 3.7), created by Gloria Willcox, can help you identify words that correlate with what you are feeling. In the middle are six primary emotions: three positive (Peaceful, Powerful and Joyful) and three difficult (Sad, Mad and Scared.) The outer two rings list secondary emotions, or how you may feel about those primary emotions. Note the blank boxes on the outer rings. These connote that even this extensive list is not exhaustive and you may have and use more descriptive words for the emotions you are feeling. The ability to identify your inner parts by either an image, name, or preferably both, is a key step toward empowering your Surface Self to work with and lead your hidden inner parts.

As you identify each inner part, ask it to step into one of many holding rooms in your submersible. These are specially designed rooms with one-way mirrors that allow you to see the part, but keep it safely separated from your observing Surface Self. Sometimes a part may refuse or feel strongly threatened when you try to place it in one of these holding rooms. Whatever the reason, the holding room analogy is not absolutely necessary. Ask the part to move to a large open platform or deck if you want. Like the holding room, the platform has a large protective barrier with a one-way mirror that separates you and the part, but allows you to still see it. This process of isolating your various emotions or parts into their separate holding spaces differentiates or separates your Surface Self from your various emotions. This prevents you from becoming overwhelmed by the emotion, thereby allowing you to rationally and calmly assess what it needs and how it is trying to serve you. We will discuss how to do that a little later.

THE FEELING WHEEL

BY GLORIA WILCOX

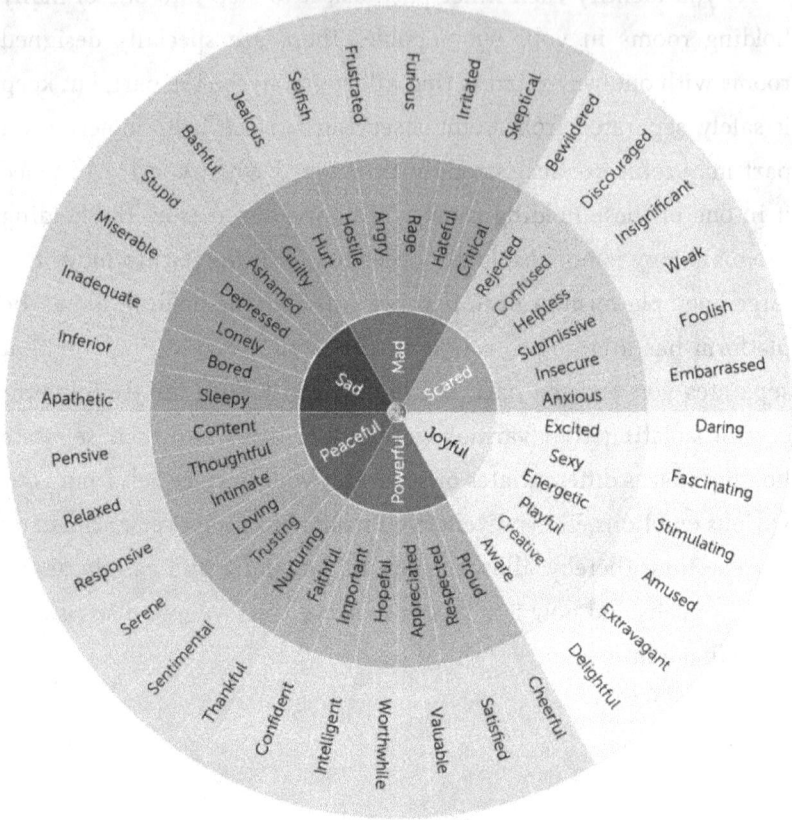

(FIGURE 3.7)

Once you have identified as many difficult emotions and parts as you can, repeat that entire process, but this time visualize a positive experience.

Modify the analogy in whatever way you need to make it work for you. If the whole underwater/exploration/submersible analogy is getting in your way, drop it. The main concept is to safely isolate your emotional parts both from each other and from your experiencing Surface Self, thus allowing you to more rationally analyze them later.

Don't think you must identify all your inner parts in a single session. I am still discovering parts of me and the unique roles they play years into my journey. How you experience your inner parts and how you imagine them will likely also morph over time. As you repeat this process and identify new parts, or as new parts of yourself spontaneously identify themselves in real life experiences, add them to your list.

I found that collecting all these images into a single collage helps me unify my assorted parts and inner characters. To help you do this, download and print a copy of the Modular Mind image from www. DrYou.org/resources. As you identify your Surface Self and your Deep Inner parts, paste your Surface Self image on the center of the Surface Brain and paste each of your inner parts images onto the area labeled Deep Brain. Now—meet the wonderful complex person called you. How does that feel? Does it feel truer than thinking of yourself as a single simple character?

3. Separate Stubborn Blended Parts

When you think you have identified as many emotions and inner characters as you can, run through a body scan one last time to see if there are any stragglers. If a part gets left behind, it's no big deal. Now that you know how to safely enter this world, you can do so whenever and as often as you want to identify any new emotions/characters/parts.

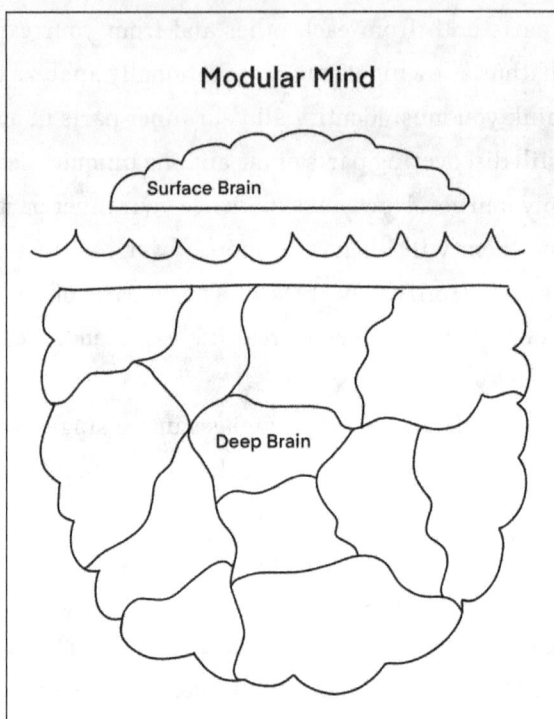

Modular Mind

Surface Brain

Deep Brain

(FIGURE 3.8)

You may feel a little overwhelmed or fearful as you think about facing your newly identified difficult emotions and parts. Remember the Compassionate Meditation tool. It will help you maintain strong, safe self-leadership. Take a few deep breaths as you need. Validate your fear or discomfort. Remind yourself that everybody experiences similar difficulties. Reassure yourself with soothing touch and comforting words as you need. Remember that you placed each part in a strong, safe space which will keep them from blending with or overwhelming your observing Surface Self. Those protective walls and see-through mirrors allow you to titrate how much of the emotion you experience.

Pick the first part or emotion you want to discover more about. Walk over to the holding room where you placed that part. While standing safely on the outside, look through the one-way mirror at the form or character that this inner part has assumed. Begin by asking, "How do I feel toward the part in the room?" If you feel something other than curiosity and compassion, find the part that is interfering and ask it to separate from your Self and step into its own holding room.

Let's use my inner characters as an example. Let's say I'm looking at the little crying boy that I identified earlier as my vulnerable, sad inner part. If I feel angry toward it while I'm looking at it from outside the holding room, my angry Monster part is interfering. I need to ask it to separate and go to its own holding room. Remember, by default your Surface Self experiences only compassion and curiosity. If you feel something other than that, some other part has blended with your observing Surface Self. Sometimes multiple parts may have remained blended simultaneously with your Surface Self, such as anger, sadness or jealousy. Repeat this step of separating each until you feel compassionate and curious enough to safely proceed.

4. Engage Parts As You Feel Comfortable

Another benefit of this tool is that it helps you control how intensely you feel the part or emotion in the holding room by how closely you engage it. You can remain on the outside of the holding room with the full protection of the steel wall and thick glass. You can unlatch the door, but stand safely in the doorway. You can enter the room, but remain distanced, or you can fully embrace that part. Progress at your own pace.

As you feel more comfortable, you will eventually want to enter the room and engage your inner part. As you do this, monitor your observing Self to make sure it is not blending with the part. Also make sure no other dysfunctional parts slip into the room and blend with your Surface Self.

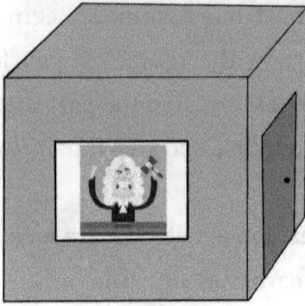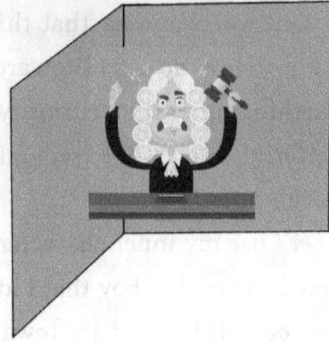

(FIGURE 3.9A)   (FIGURE 3.9B)

If you feel anything other than compassion and curiosity, stop, calm your body if needed, identify the blending part, and ask it to go to its own holding room. Assure it that after dealing with this first part, you will visit it and provide whatever it needs.

If you need to leave the room and come back later, remember your observing Surface Self is in control. For this visualization process to be most successful, you want your observing Self to remain fully differentiated from your various inner characters and parts.

5. Identify Common Dysfunctional Roles

Each inner character represents a discrete part of you that functions in a specific role. Each has its own worldview, interests, beliefs, feelings, and ways of expressing itself. It is autonomous, yet lives within the society of your Deep System and interacts with and engages your other inner characters. When the various parts of your brain work in harmony, they all operate as a unified whole, a single collective functional unit. When this happens, you become lost in the moment and don't notice the individual parts. Everything fades into the background except the task at hand. This frequently happens to me when I read an interesting novel, play my guitar or speed down a beautiful section of single track on my mountain bike. Think back to an experience when you were lost in something you really enjoyed doing. Close your eyes and picture it. What did it feel like? Dr. Mihaly Csikszentmihalyi calls these moments "Flow."[33] He contends that we feel happiest and most content when we work in this harmonious flow state. We will talk more about flow in the chapter on Assets.

Unfortunately, like every other human system in our outer world, the characters of your deep inner system don't always work harmoniously. When the leaders of organizations don't guide their staff effectively, adversity often causes the company to descend into chaos. Individuals are forced to do the best they can to resolve the problem with their own limited skills and perspective. Without the benefits of an effective leader, a master plan and all the needed skills, individuals produce ineffective solutions.

Similarly, without effective leadership from your internal leader—your Surface Self—adversity commonly forces your Deep Self's characters to assume responsibility for keeping you safe by taking on protective roles. None of your individual deep parts possesses all the skills to do the job effectively. The results are skewed. As I mentioned earlier in this chapter, this is similar to someone singing out of tune. Their discordant efforts stand out and automatically draw your attention to the problem. That is the purpose of strong difficult emotions. They focus your attention and motivate you to change something.

These protective roles assumed by your inner characters are not the natural roles for which they were originally designed, therefore they are considered dysfunctional, burdened or polarized roles. Your inner parts would prefer not to assume these burdened roles, but feel they have no choice. As discord breaks out and parts become polarized, you will experience inner turmoil.

---

33   Mialy Csikszentmihalyi, *Flow: The Psychology of Optimal Experience* (Harper Perennial Modern Classics, 2008).

Dr. Schartz defines twelve common dysfunctional roles that inner characters assume.[34]

1. **The Exiled:** The most sensitive parts. They are often viewed as child-like inner parts and described as sad, weak and vulnerable. When you are injured or outraged, your system often buries them in deep bunkers to prevent them from being felt or acknowledged. Like the character Sadness in *Inside Out*, these exiles will expand until you pay attention.

2. **Striver:** Uses achievement, success, wealth, and power to distract. Often it is highly critical.

3. **Hyper-aroused Sentry or warrior:** Stays on continuous danger alert, constantly feeling like it is in jeopardy, leaving you with a continual sense of anxiety.

4. **Perfectionist/Pleaser:** Attempts to do everything perfectly and please everyone so they will not be abandoned.

5. **Passive Pessimist:** Tries to avoid interpersonal risk by making the Self apathetic and withdrawn so they won't get too close to anyone.

6. **Inner Terrorist:** Assumes the role of an abuser who scares the weaker inner characters into submission.

7. **Controller:** Driven by an obsessive need to intellectually solve problems, it pushes aside all feelings.

8. **Caretaker:** Always sacrifices its personal needs to focus on the care of others.

9. **Entitled One:** Encourages the Self to pursue whatever it wants no matter who is injured or wronged.

---

34 Richard Schwartz, *Internal Family Systems Therapy*, (The Guilford Press, 1997).

10. **Dependent One:** Keeps the Self in a victim role to ensure others will take care of them.

11. **Denier:** Distorts perceptions, keeps you from seeing and responding to risky feedback.

12. **Firefighter:** If the exiled parts break loose, filling you with profound hurt or sadness and none of the other roles control the discomfort, part of you may reach out to your destructive, unhealthy, addictive behaviors. Like firefighters who automatically take action to extinguish fires, these parts automatically take action to extinguish your pain with your favorite numbing activities.

How well your inner parts interact and the roles they assume depends partially on your genetics and partially on the environment you were exposed to while your brain was still forming. In individuals whose mood setpoint or explanatory style falls in the spectrum of pessimism, your parts will assume dysfunctional roles more easily. In addition, when you are chronically exposed to more intense adversity, your inner characters are more likely to assume dysfunctional roles. These adversarial roles destroy the cohesiveness and harmony of your deep inner system.

Unfortunately, people develop most of their chronic coping strategies when they are young, more vulnerable to external environments (primary caretakers) and when they poorly understand how to release their own natural self-leadership resources. The results are entrenched automatic dysfunctional coping strategies that they carry into adulthood. Most of us never know any better, so we accept our lot in life and live in a state of chronic overwhelm.

The good news is that there is a better way. It is worth the time and effort to explore your inner characters and map their interactions. When your parts don't think your Surface Self is paying attention to them or that your Surface Self has the leadership skills to meet their needs, they will continue to assume protective yet dysfunctional roles. The role a part plays will shift depending on the situation. Notice in the list below, my Happy Playful Boy plays multiple parts.

If you identify any dysfunctional role a part is playing, write that down beside the image of your inner part or in a separate list of your inner parts.

My Inner Parts as an Example:

Thomas Edison
Role: Striver

Dr. Spock
Role: Controller

Hippy
Role: Denier

Sad Boy
Role: Exiled (same character as Happy Boy: when one is exiled so is the other)

Happy Playful Boy
Role: Exiled/Firefighter/Denier

Angry Monster
Role: Firefighter/Inner Terrorist

Judge
Role: Perfectionist

Mother Teresa
Role: Caretaker

Chameleon
Role: Pleaser

6. Discover Underlying Needs

Once you have identified a part's dysfunctional role or coping strategies, the next step is to uncover its underlying need. Ask why it has assumed such a dysfunctional, polarized role.

Dr. Schwarz and his colleagues recommend that you start by asking questions similar to these.

1. Why are you doing or saying [extreme behavior or thought]?

2. What do you really want?

3. What are you afraid will happen if you stop doing or saying [extreme behavior or thought]?

4. If the Surface Self were able to lead effectively and keep [the feared consequence] from happening, so you could do anything you want in the system, what would you do?

5. Would you like help in this new role?

The Five Whys

Sometimes, the answer you get points to a deeper hidden need. I like to drill down to the core of an issue by using the Five Whys Method. Starting with your initial answer, ask, "Why?" Repeat asking "Why?" with each subsequent answer until you discover the core answer. Typically, by the fifth "Why," you have your real answer.

Example:

Cheryl was struggling with an Angry part that recently responded hostilely to her best friend when she didn't promptly return Cheryl's phone call.

First Why: She asked her Angry part, "Why did you do that?"
Her Angry part replied: "Because that wasn't very considerate of her."

Second Why: "Why do you think that wasn't very considerate?"
Its reply: "Because a true friend would have cared enough to call back in a timely manner."

Third Why: "Why do you feel it is important for a friend to call back in a timely manner?"
Its reply: "Because that shows respect."

Fourth Why: "Why is respect so important to you?"
Its reply: "Because respect shows they care."

Fifth Why: "Why is it important for others to show they care."
Its reply: "Because when they don't, I feel worthless or unworthy of their love."

Now we understand the problem or the underlying Core Negative Belief and its associated Fundamental Need. We'll discuss how to address Core Negative Beliefs in the next chapter. Cheryl feels unworthy of love. Anger has assumed the dysfunctional, burdened role of an aggressive Sentry. This Sentry feels it must assertively protect Cheryl from feeling worthless or unloved. It had tried to communicate to Cheryl that she needed to lead in a more assertive and clear way that honored her need to feel loved and cared for. More effective self-leadership would clearly communicate this sense of feeling unloved when her friend doesn't call her back in a timely manner. Her angry part then would not feel the need to play the part of an overly aggressive Sentry.

I mentioned earlier that we all have basic needs that must be met for us to function at our best. These fundamental needs are not merely wants or desires. Various researchers call them different things and don't always agree on the exact number, but—as a reminder—we all have nine fundamental needs: affection, autonomy and freedom, inclusion, security, identity, meaningful work, sustenance (food, water, shelter), mastery, and rest/recovery. As you identify a part's underlying needs, write it down beside the dysfunctional role the part is assuming. Some parts may have several needs. You may use different words or identify needs that I did not list. That's fine. Use whatever word best expresses what the part is telling you it needs. Also note that the need of a part may change with time.

My inner parts as an example:

Thomas Edison
Role: Striver
Need: Inclusion, Affection/Worthiness, Identity, Meaningful Work

Dr. Spock
Role: Controller
Need: Mastery, Affection, Identity, Meaningful Work

Hippy
Role: Denier
Need: Freedom

Sad Boy
Role: Exiled
Need: Affection, Autonomy, Inclusion

Happy Playful Boy
Role: Exiled/Firefighter/Denier
Need: Affection, Rest/Recovery/Recreation, Inclusion

Angry Monster
Role: Firefighter/Inner Terrorist
Need: Security/Safety, Affection

Judge
Role: Perfectionist
Need: Mastery, Affection/Worthiness

Mother Teresa
Role: Caretaker
Need: Affection, Meaningful Work

Chameleon
Role: Pleaser
Need: Affection

Now go back to the part and assure it that your Surface Self will lead and provide for it effectively. Thank it for its efforts and release it from its dysfunctional, burdened role.

Sometimes a part will need more time and reassurance. It will release its burdened role only when it firmly believes that your Surface Self has learned to listen to it and protect it.

Before leaving the topic of dysfunctional roles, I want to address the fact that positive emotions or parts can also play dysfunctional roles. In *Inside Out*, Joy comes to the realization that she has ironically played a role in Riley's depression. Whenever Riley's inner part, Sadness, begins to express itself, Joy feels the need to step in and do something to suppress it. We do this when we engage in addictive, feel-good behaviors, as we discussed earlier. Instead of allowing ourselves to feel the discomfort of the moment, we sweep in with retail therapy, sex, drugs, alcohol, overworking or social media. Because of Joy's constant attempt to suppress Sadness, Sadness feels unheard. As a result, it intensifies its voice until Riley can no longer ignore it.

Perpetual happiness or optimism is not realistic and the pursuit of it is actually destructive. A healthier approach requires allowing ourselves to experience all of our emotions in safe, non-overwhelming ways. When those hurting parts feel heard and understood, they transform into much less menacing versions of themselves.

7. Watch Your Inner Parts Transform

If you have chronically suppressed and numbed difficult emotions, just separating your Surface Self from your various Deep Parts is a huge step even if you don't initially enter any of the holding rooms. Allowing yourself to experience your deep inner parts at any differentiated state is a major positive step. Congratulate yourself and celebrate your progress. As you safely revisit your newly differentiated deep emotions, try to get closer than the time before until you can finally communicate openly with them.

As your deep emotions take on healthier roles, your view of them will change. They will morph or transform into something that better represents their new role. As I mentioned earlier, one of my strong resistant characters was the Angry Monster. As I relinquished my Angry part from the primary role of protecting me, I watched it morph from a dangerous-looking monster into a respectful guard who stood watch and protected my personal boundaries. As you did when you initially identified your inner parts, pay close attention to what this newly transformed part looks like. Sketch an image of it or find a picture that best represents it. Now pull out your Modular Mind sheet and paste this newly transformed image over the old part.

Before I leave the topic of personal boundaries, I want to clarify what I mean by that. Personal boundaries can be thought of as guidelines, rules or limits that a person creates to identify reasonable, safe and permissible ways for other people to behave toward you. They also establish healthy ways with which you can respond when someone crosses those boundaries. My new healthy boundaries look a lot like the US and Canadian border. They are respectful and porous enough to allow friendly people to pass through—thus allowing close, meaningful relationships—while firm enough to prevent caustic people from taking advantage of me.

During this transition state, your protective inner character's automatic reactions may initially intensify. They will eventually relinquish control only once you prove to them that you can consistently keep yourself safe and healthy. Before they agree to fully relinquish their protective roles, however, you may get them to agree to use less scary and destructive behaviors.

I have described DCE in vivid detail as a symbolic underwater exploratory process. As I said earlier, if the underwater analogy doesn't resonate with you, drop it. It is only a tool. The most important part of the process is to safely separate your observing self from your various emotional parts, identify their underlying needs and effectively meet those needs. If another analogy works better for you, use it.

Other possible analogies to consider are:

Surface Self	Deep Self
Director	Cast of Characters
Coach	Team/Players
Captain	Crew
Chief	Tribe
Foreman	Workers
CEO	Employees
Conductor	Orchestra
President/Prime Minister	Congress/House of Commons

As an example, with the Coach/Team model, you could similarly envision your observing self as a coach who remotely analyzes video footage of their inner deep players as they perform their unique roles during a game.

Both of Dr. Schwartz's books, *Internal Family Systems Therapy* and *You Are the One You've Been Waiting For*, are good resources if you want to pursue this process more deeply. As always, if you find this overwhelming or you're still struggling and need more help, I recommend that you reach out to a good therapist, counselor or psychologist.

Summary

1. Overconsumption of good feeling behaviors overly stimulates dopamine leading to decreased dopamine release and downregulation of dopamine receptors.

2. All emotions are good when viewed as part of a system that is meant to protect you, like the various colored lights of a traffic signal.

3. Awareness involves listening to and allowing yourself to experience the full gamut of emotions, both positive and difficult.

4. Emotions alert you first in the body and can most easily be dampened at this level.

5. Four ways to embrace your emotions (listed from simplest to most revealing):

   a. Three Ds: Discontinue, Distance, Distract

   b. Mountaintop Observer

   c. Compassionate Meditation

   d. Deep Character Exploration (DCE)

As you have discovered, **Awareness** is about recognizing the initial response of emotions in your body and learning to manage them in healthy ways. The next step in the stress response system, after the body's response, is for the MPFC (Medial Prefrontal Cortex) of the Surface Brain to become activated. Here, you finally become consciously aware of your emotions as thoughts.

Sometimes your best efforts to recognize your emotions in your body and control them are not as successful as you may wish. When this happens, your difficult emotions can produce automatic unhelpful, stressful thoughts. The next chapter, **Attenuation**, identifies several ways you can dampen these automatic unhealthy ways of thinking.

CHAPTER 4

Attenuation — Dispute Your Automatic Negative Thoughts

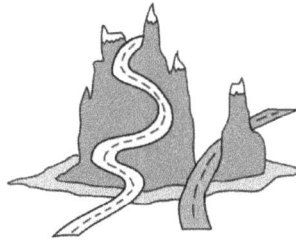

ARRIVAL GATE 1A: Adversity

DEPARTURE GATE 6A: Awareness, Attenuation, Assets, Allies, Aim, Action

Boarding Pass	Empowered Self-Care	Boarding Pass
Username: _____ **First Class**		← ✈ Departures
Destination: Beautiful Life Current Location: Reality		✈ 6A
Arrival: **Gate 1A** (Adversity)		Gate
Departure: **Gate 6A** (Awareness, Attenuation, Assets, Allies, Aim, Action)		

Most people think: they want their difficult thoughts
to completely disappear.

The truth is: our difficult thoughts represent something good and beautiful about us. A more constructive approach is to embrace these difficult thoughts while attenuating them to healthier levels.

"Excellence is an art won by training and habituation [...] We are what we repeatedly do. Excellence, then, is not an act, but a habit."[35]

"For as he thinketh in his heart, so is he."[36]

"All that we are is the result of what we have thought: it is founded on our thoughts and is made up of thoughts."[37]

Automatic Thoughts and Thinking Errors

Your brain's Deep System uses shortcuts to help it process large quantities of information efficiently, quickly and effortlessly. These automatic shortcuts are often referred to as heuristics. They allow you to focus your more limited conscious attention on the most important tasks while your Deep Brain runs everything else automatically and effortlessly in the background. Without heuristics, your conscious Surface Brain would become overwhelmed with the sheer volume of tasks to be done. Heuristics also help you make decisions when information is scant and when speed is more important than accuracy. Despite all their good, however, you can pay for their automaticity and speed in the form of processing errors, or what psychologists call cognitive distortions.

Heuristics act like spam filters on your computer that identify "unimportant" email messages. Most of the time these filters work well, but occasionally important messages get sent to your junk

---

35 Aristotle, https://www.forbes.com/quotes/659/.

36 Proverbs 23.7.

37 Thomas Byrom, *Dhammapada: The sayings of the Buddha* (Shambhala, 1993).

folder. While fast and efficient, your Deep System's shortcuts can also introduce similar inaccurate distorted ways of thinking.

So far you've learned how the human brain initially arrives at troubled destinations or becomes overwhelmed as it processes **Adversity**. This then led to the question, "How do I get out of here?" In Chapter 3, you began the six-part process of departing from difficult mental destinations by exploring your emotions through **Awareness**. In this second part, you will learn ways to **Attenuate** or dispute your automatic unhealthy thinking patterns or cognitive distortions.

Beauty in the Turbulence

In 2020, our youngest child graduated from high school. Her graduation marked not only a significant transition in her life, but also in the life of my wife and myself. We were becoming empty-nesters. This called for a celebration, but like everybody else in the world, the COVID pandemic altered our original plans. Instead of jumping on a jet bound for Europe, we packed into our fifth wheel RV, which my wife calls "Ha-**RV**-ey," and set off to explore the Grand Canyon.

I had never been to the Grand Canyon, and as with most first-time visitors I was struck by its immense size and hostile beauty. In many ways, it represents the rugged mentality and fierce independence of the earlier settlers who forged west and founded the United States.

As I reflected on the scene before me, I pondered the turmoil in the world—the pandemic, civil unrest and political infighting. The canyon below was a beautiful metaphor of how we frequently lock ourselves into unhealthy automatic ways of thinking.

Water flows passively or automatically downhill. The Colorado River, which runs through the Grand Canyon, begins as melting snow high in the peaks of the Rocky Mountains and flows some 1,450 miles to the Gulf of Colorado in Mexico between the Baja peninsula and Sonora.

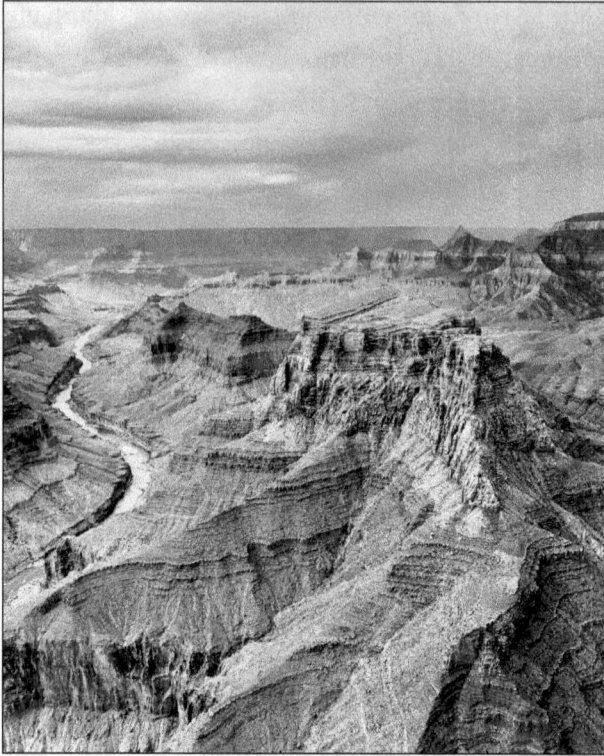

(FIGURE 4.1)[38]

Along its course, it drops two vertical miles, thirty times steeper than the Mississippi River. The combination of steep gradient and narrow canyons creates some of the largest and most violent rapids in the world. As the powerful, rumbling mixture of water and sediment flows through the canyon, it continuously excavates its own channel, digging deeper and deeper into the surrounding rock. With every cubic foot of water, the river becomes more defined and ensnared by its own steep cliffs. It creates a deep predestined path that leaves the river little choice but to surge in a single direction. It constrains and

---

38   Haley Ball, Colorado River in Grand Canyon, 2020.

enslaves itself through its own passive and automatic actions. Feel familiar? Your thinking can do the same thing.

Attitudes, behaviors, assumptions, and thought patterns often follow a similar passive course through your Deep Brain. Like the water of the Colorado River, every time you think or behave the neural channels that flow through your brain become more entrenched and defined. Obviously, they don't cut physical channels in your brain, but the neural pathways become more efficient at transmitting signals. Myelin, an insulator that wraps nerve pathways, serves a similar function as rubber does around electrical wires. When neural pathways are repetitively used, your brain believes these attitudes, behaviors and thought patterns are important, so it optimizes their transmission. One way it does this is by thickening the myelin around them. Your brain also achieves greater efficiency by increasing the number of connection points between sequential neurons.

Given enough time, these pathways become so efficient that they propagate automatically; they require no intentional thought or initiation on your part. Riding a bike, recognizing written words, typing, and spontaneous emotional responses are all examples of automatic neural pathways. As I mentioned at the beginning of this chapter, automaticity produces efficiency and speed, but like the tumultuous rapids of the Colorado, automatic thinking can also create unseen dangers.

The most fierce and powerful rapids lie in the deepest part of the Grand Canyon, where the cliffs are vertical and the passage is narrow. Your automatic neural processes—the swiftest, most entrenched and potentially most dangerous—also lie within the deepest part of your brain, well below your sense of awareness. As with the hidden dangers of rapids, automatic thinking processes can silently lead to unhealthy, dangerous places.

Common Types of Distorted Automatic Negative Thoughts

Over the last couple of decades, psychologists have identified and categorized the most common distorted Automatic Negative Thoughts (ANTs), also called Cognitive Distortions.

- **Mind Reading (MR):** You believe you understand what people are thinking without sufficient evidence to support that belief.

- **Fortune Telling (FT):** You predict events in the future will unfold negatively with little evidence to support your assumptions.

- **Catastrophizing (C):** You emphasize the worst possible outcomes.

- **Labeling (L):** You attach generalized negative traits to yourself and others.

- **Discounting Positives (DP):** You feel that positive traits of yourself and others are trivial.

- **Negative Bias (NB):** You focus almost exclusively on negatives. This blinds you seeing the positives and recognizing opportunities.

- **Overgeneralizing (OG):** You extrapolate a negative bias to all circumstances based on a singular event.

- **All-Or-Nothing Thinking (AON):** This is also called Dichotomous Thinking. You see a problem either one way or another and fail to recognize the many nuances that may have contributed to the situation.

- **Shoulds (S):** You focus on how things "should" be instead of how they are.

- **Personalizing (P):** You believe you are disproportionately responsible for negative events and fail to see other potential causes.

- **Blaming (B):** You believe external sources are the origin of your problems and fail to take responsibility for your part.

- **Unfair Comparisons (UC):** You assign an unrealistic standard to yourself, others and circumstances.

- **Regret Orientation (RO):** You focus on what you could have done better in the past instead of trying to do the best you can now.

- **What If (WI):** You continuously worry that you, others and circumstances will fail to meet your expectations.

- **Emotional Reasoning (ER):** You let your feelings guide your decisions or interpretation of people, events and circumstances.

- **Inability to Disconfirm (ID):** You reject any evidence or arguments that might contradict your preconceived negative beliefs.

- **Judgment Focus (JF):** You evaluate all things as either good or bad rather than simply describing, accepting or understanding. Judgment thinking is a particularly destructive form of dichotomous thinking.[39]

Later in the chapter, we will discuss how to identify your own distorted thoughts. In the following sections, we'll get acquainted with several ways of attenuating your difficult emotions.

Writing: Your Primary Tool for Exploration and Discovery

Because automatic thinking errors occur in the background of your subconscious Deep Brain, you may not realize they are occurring

---

39 Robert L. Leahy, Stepehn J. F. Holland, and Lata K. McGinn, *Treatment Plans and Interventions for Depression and Anxiety Disorders, Second Edition* (The Guilford Press, 2000)

when they initially start. Writing is one of the best ways to bring these errors to consciousness so you can recognize their distortions and learn how to dispute them.

According to James W. Pennebaker, PhD, leading researcher on expressive writing and author of *Opening Up by Writing It Down*, there are several reasons why writing helps you process your thoughts.

1. Writing slows your thinking. This provides space and time for you to explore possible links between seemingly disparate thoughts and experiences. By slowing down, you are more likely to recognize potentially powerful revelations.

2. Writing involves a physical component which engages more areas of your brain, thus boosting your cognitive power.

3. Writing expands your search windows. Humans naturally look for links and patterns in our experiences. Your attention, however, naturally focuses on information and experiences that you recall more easily. Thus, you place more emphasis on things that happened recently and events that are associated with strong emotions. Writing helps expand your search to information that may not be so easily remembered. Think back to a time when you reread notes you took during a lecture. How often do you rediscover important pieces of information that you forgot the speaker said?

4. Writing helps you evaluate options more thoroughly. Humans have a bias toward simple answers. If an easy-to-understand answer makes sense, people often stop looking for other explanations, even though more complex answers may better explain the situation.

5. Writing makes information more difficult to ignore. Humans are good at failing to notice helpful cause-and-effect relationships

because we simply don't want to see them. Once on paper, they are harder to ignore.

6. Writing frees up mental energy to do more positive, constructive work. It requires energy to suppress things you don't want to see. As you free up mental energy, you become more creative and insightful, therefore better able to understand and assimilate confusing information.

7. Writing helps you translate into words what your Deep Brain is feeling. Your Surface Brain, the part of your brain that constructs and implements practical plans to solve your distressing problems, understands words better than feelings.

8. Writing helps you break the perpetual circuit of negative ruminations. Once your Surface Brain formulates a plan of action, your Deep Brain feels free to release you from recurring negative thoughts.

Mood Journaling

Mood Journaling is a portion of a more comprehensive writing strategy that I use for self-leadership and self-care. I'll discuss this comprehensive journaling structure in the Aim chapter. However, for now we will focus on the mood journaling section to explore and attenuate difficult emotions and thoughts.

This writing strategy is a self-directed, more simplified version of Cognitive Behavioral Therapy (CBT) that many therapists use. Even if you are not ready to commit to mood journaling, studies show that simply reading about how to practice CBT can help. As always, if you find this process overwhelming, I encourage you to find a talented therapist.

In the Mood Journaling process I use, there are five steps:

1. Record your difficult emotions.
2. Record the associated negative thoughts.
3. Rate their intensity.
4. Assign a new healthy goal.
5. **Attenuate** with the Sword of Truth.

    A: Alternatives

    E: Evidence

    I: Implications

    O: Observe

    U: Usefulness

6. Reassess the intensity of your emotions and associated negative thoughts.

If you want a downloadable copy of my Mood Journal template (Figure 4.2), go to www.DrYou.org/resources. Use it as is, modify it, or develop your own. If you develop your own helpful or fun version, share it with us. Your version may resonate with somebody more than mine does or it might encourage others to develop their own adaptation.

1. Record your difficult emotions

Building on what you learned in the last chapter, record the difficult emotions that you identified there and continue to identify as you encounter new challenges.

As you work with your difficult emotions, remember to keep your observing self separated and at a healthy distance from them. If you feel your difficult emotions blending with your observing self, go back to the Mountaintop Observer, Compassionate Mediation or DCE tools and work with the emotion until you feel safe to proceed.

2. Record Your Automatic Negative Thoughts

Beneath each difficult emotion, list all the automatic negative thoughts you tell yourself as you experience them. Record these thoughts exactly as you tell them to yourself. Don't edit them. Use the language you may never use in public, but that you regularly use with yourself. This is the time to be completely honest. Nobody is going to see these entries unless you decide to share them.

If you identified any Core Negative Beliefs in the previous chapter, list them here as well. If you haven't tried it yet, for each difficult emotion and set of associated automatic negative emotions use the Five Whys strategy from the last chapter to see if you can discover an underlying Core Negative Belief.

Date:	
Record your difficult emotions:	
Record the associated negative thoughts:	
Rate their intensities (0-100):	
Assign a new healthy goal (0-100):	
Attenuate: Alternatives Evidence Implications Observe Usefulness	
Reassess their intensities (0-100):	
Common Cognitive Distortions	Mind Reading, Fortune Telling, Catastrophizing, Labeling, Discounting the Positives, Negativity Bias, Over Generalization, All-or-None Thinking, Shoulds, Self Blaming, Blaming Others, Unfair Comparisons, Regret Orientation, What Ifs, Emotional Reasoning, Inability to Disconfirm

(FIGURE 4.2)

3. Rate the intensity

Rate the intensity of your difficult emotions and associated automatic negative thoughts on a scale from 0-100.

4. Assign new, healthy goals

Do you believe you shouldn't feel your current pain? Do you want to make your difficult emotions and negative thoughts magically disappear? If so, think about this. Your difficult emotions and negative thoughts contain positive information about your needs and values; they reveal something good and special about you. If you could magically make them disappear, you would also lose touch with those positive aspects of yourself. That may not be something you want to do. An alternative to erasing or obliterating your difficult emotions and negative thoughts is to attenuate them to less threatening levels. Remember, each of your emotions is similar to a light in a traffic signal. Each light works as a part of a larger system and is dependent on the others to help protect you. If you destroy the red lights, green lights become meaningless.

As a broad continuum of feelings, your emotions create a scale you use to assign value to yourself and your external world. Without the full range of all your emotions, the scale becomes useless. If you destroy difficult emotions, you're left with a group of random feelings that have no context. You're not left with happiness. You're left with numbness, a world devoid of a functional emotional system. Does that sound like a world in which you would want to live?

Similarly, your automatic negative thoughts and your underlying core negative beliefs also contain information that point to positive qualities about you, your positive core values and your strengths.

Let's look at Charles. Charles works in a high-pressure outdoor sales position. Historically, he has been one of his company's top salespeople. His unrelenting work ethic and desire to do everything perfectly has always served him well at work, but is causing problems at home. He works 10-13 hours a day, six days a week, leaving little time and energy to devote to his family. When he is home, his relationships suffer because of his harsh criticism. A few months ago, the fighting between him and his wife became so bad that he moved out of the house. He admits he doesn't want to get a divorce, but can't seem to make it work.

In the past, work served as a refuge from the turmoil at home. More recently, however, stress at work mounted as the economy declined. Several of his larger clients canceled their orders and new customers have been more difficult than usual to find. Two weeks ago, Charles's boss told him that unless his sales numbers improved, he would be let go.

Charles initially presented to my office complaining of abdominal bloating and irregular bowel movements, alternating between constipation and diarrhea. His initial exam and tests were all normal. He said the symptoms weren't severe enough to warrant a prescription, so we discussed boosting natural sources of fiber in his diet and starting a probiotic.

A couple of weeks later, he returned with the same symptoms. This time I inquired about stressors at home or work, and he admitted he was about to lose both his job and his wife. He couldn't understand why after working so hard, he was about to lose it all.

I asked him to write down his most disturbing recurrent difficult thoughts. He said he kept telling himself, "I always screw up everything. I can never do anything right." While concentrating on those thoughts, I asked him, "If those thoughts could point to something good about yourself, what would they be?" Initially he couldn't think of anything, so I asked him to close his eyes, take a few slow deep breaths and concentrate on a scenario when he had succeeded or done something well. He said he could picture a time when he ran a fundraiser for a local charity. He was the only person who would volunteer and, as usual, he applied his hard, driving work style to the task and raised more money in a single fundraiser than had ever been raised.

Thinking back on his previous statements, he realized his harsh self-criticisms were a reflection of how deeply he cares and his high standards. I reminded him that if he erased every trace of those self-critical thoughts, he would also erase those positive qualities. He agreed that those positive qualities were not aspects of himself that he was willing to lose.

Because you probably don't want to delete all that is good and right about yourself either, a better strategy is to reduce difficult emotions and negative thoughts to more tolerable levels. Instead of an on-off switch, think about using a sliding toggle that works much like a see-saw. When you reduce one side (the difficult emotions and thoughts), the other side (positive emotions and thoughts) automatically elevates.

Using this sliding toggle analogy, I want you to go back to your list of difficult emotions and negative thoughts and assign an intensity level (0-100) that feels more acceptable—something that feels safer and less overwhelming, but still allows the emotion or thought to exist. Instead of zero, this will now become your new target goal for your difficult emotion or thought. Record that new intensity goal in your mood journal.

Instead of obliterating your difficult emotions and thoughts, you have now started the process of **Attenuating** or reducing them to more manageable levels. Notice that as you change the objective from obliterating to attenuating, you automatically adopt a more curious and non-judgmental mindset toward those emotions and thoughts. Curiosity fosters exploration. Safe exploration generates new discoveries about your underlying hidden needs and healthier ways to provide for those needs. The path to healing runs directly through the heart of your difficult emotions and thoughts. Attenuated levels allow you to embrace them and experience them in safe ways that foster curious exploration. If you suppress them or allow yourself to experience their discomfort, you bypass them and miss the path of discovery that they reveal. The bottom line is that we must embrace the discomfort to move forward. Dr. Robert Leahy, clinical professor of psychiatry and author of *The Worry Cure*, calls this **Constructive Discomfort,** which is similar to the discomfort we feel while exercising. The path to success for both your mind and your body runs through the middle of that constructive discomfort.

5. Attenuate with the Sword of Truth.

I call this tool the **Sword of Truth** because it cuts your difficult emotions and thoughts into more manageable sizes by undermining their toxic foundations.

According to the legend of King Arthur, his sword Excalibur held magical powers. As Merlin foretold, only the true heir to the throne could pull the sword from the stone. After many nobles tried and failed, the teenage Arthur released the sword from the stone effortlessly. Excalibur protected him and bestowed upon him great powers to rule with wisdom and valor.

"Then you will know the truth and the truth shall set you free."[40] While I can't grant you a magic sword that will make your difficult thoughts and emotions disappear, I can help you release your own natural but constrained inner strengths. Because the most fundamental power of the human Surface Brain is the ability to express concepts with language, I use the five vowels **(A, E, I, O, U),** which compose the core of the English language, to represent the key aspects of the **Attenuation** process: **Alternatives, Evidence, Implications, Observation,** and **Usefulness.** These five components, when welded together, become your greatest weapon, the **Sword of Truth.** This sword, your rational arguments, thrusts compassion and truth into the heart of your cognitive distortions and emotional lies.

---

40 John 8:32.

A. Alternatives

One of the purposes of difficult emotions and thoughts is to focus your attention on problems. It's a survival or protective effect. When a saber-toothed tiger is prowling about and you hear a twig snap in the dark, your Deep System immediately turns toward the sound. You strain with all the might of your senses to focus on the threat. As you slip on these ancient blinders, your focus becomes narrowed and you only see the perceived problem. All other issues fade into the background. With **Alternatives** you intentionally pull the blinders off and broaden your perspective.

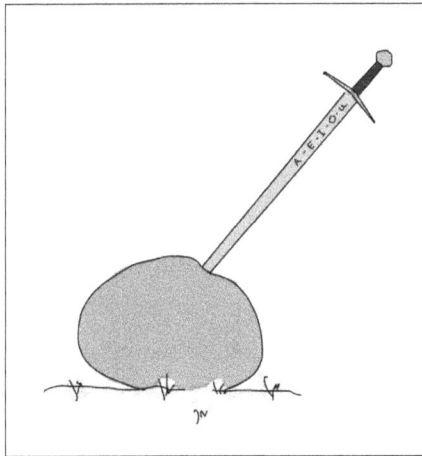

(FIGURE 4.3)

Look at one of your difficult emotions or associated negative thoughts then list as many alternative ways of thinking or feeling about your current situation as you can. It doesn't matter if you believe these alternatives are 100 percent true or that they are even very likely. All that matters is that you believe they are possible. How many alternatives can you identify? Record them in your journal.

E. Evidence

The second component of the Sword of Truth is Evidence. Draw a line down the center of a page. Above the left side write "Evidence For [your thoughts]" and above the right side, "Evidence Against." Now list all the facts you can think of to support each. Another way to think of this is a Cost/Benefit ledger. As with the above, label the top of one side of a page "Costs" and the other side "Benefits."

List all the costs and benefits of your current way of thinking. When you finish, you may want to ask a trusted friend for their input. What does the preponderance of the evidence show? Note the benefits for the way you currently think. Do those benefits outweigh the costs? Write down your thoughts.

I. Implications

In the heat of a crisis, problems often loom larger than they are. They can consume our attention and energy and shift our focus to the worst possible outcomes. This is known as catastrophizing. Changing your perspective and placing these types of problems into context can help de-escalate your runaway negative thoughts.

One way to place your situation into perspective is to list alternative outcomes that may not be as severe as the ones you are imagining. As with any type of alternative thinking, it doesn't matter if you believe it is absolutely true or even likely. The important thing is to recognize that there are other possibilities. Can you list some alternatives to the catastrophic scenarios you may be envisioning?

Another way I like to place my negative thinking into perspective is with what I call "Starry Night Therapy." I typically get up early, around 3:00 a.m.-4:00 a.m., to read, study, write, and exercise. If my thoughts are overly troublesome, I take a walk down my driveway while gazing up at the sky. I'm fortunate that on clear nights, I can see thousands of stars and even the Milky Way right outside my front door. Similarly, in my home office hangs a picture of the Milky Way my wife took while we were sitting on the rim of the Grand Canyon. Both my early morning strolls and this picture remind me that I am small and my problems are insignificant in the grand scheme of things.

Cheryl was a single mother who decided to go back to college and finish her bachelor's degree. She was finding it difficult to balance work, family and her studies. About three years ago, her husband left her for a woman with whom he was having an affair. Already struggling with a poor self-image, she recently failed a history exam which released a cascade of negative thoughts. She personalized her failure, seeing it not as a series of poor studying habits or difficulty managing her schedule, but as condemnation of herself. This failure also represented in her mind a pervasive flaw that extended into all areas of her life. And finally, she viewed the consequences of the failure as permanent. By the time I saw her, she had created a long mental road of What Ifs that ended in her not graduating and never being able to adequately support her children. This triad of personal, permanent and pervasive toxicity is the perfect recipe for depression.

One of the tools we used to help her was to de-catastrophize her depressing thoughts by challenging the implications she had created. After calming her emotions with a meditative, deep-breathing technique, I asked her to visualize her lifespan as a timeline that stretched across the length of a football field, and then to place a point on the timeline that represented this history exam. I asked her to compare that point to the rest of the timeline and to note how small it was compared to the rest of her life.

In her mind's eye, I also asked her to walk out to the point of her history exam, to stand there and look to her future. What could her life look like if she changed her perspective about failure and viewed it as a learning experience that could propel her forward, rather than as a condemnation of her character? I asked her to imagine that better version of her life, even if she didn't necessarily believe it was 100 percent possible. While continuing to visualize herself standing on that point, I asked her to imagine what her life would look like if she continued to see all her failures as permanent, personal and pervasive. I asked her to contrast the two and then write about those thoughts in her journal. I finally asked her how important on a scale of 0-10 was it for her to live into that better version of her life. She replied that it was a ten, so I asked her why not a five. It wasn't a five because she desperately wanted to provide a better life for her children. This reason was more important than any I could have given her.

Think about your own life as a long timeline and whatever struggle you are experiencing as a dot on that line, or visualize your life as speck in the great starry night. Walk through the questions I asked Cheryl and record your answers in your journal. How important is it for you to achieve a better version of your future?

O. Observe

"O" is your old friend, the Mountaintop Observer. Because I covered this in the last chapter, I'm only going to briefly mention it here. Take a few deep breaths and imagine yourself climbing to the peak of a mountain, leaving all your emotions and difficult thoughts down in the river valley below. As each emotion and thought floats into your consciousness like a leaf or boat on the river, allow yourself to experience them at this safe distance. Learn from them. Listen to what they say. Are they productive? If so, take corrective action. If unproductive, simply experience them until they float out of sight.

U. Usefulness

How do you know when to let difficult emotions and thoughts flow by and when to listen to them? Asked another way: how can you identify an emotion or thought as productive vs. unproductive? Do your difficult emotions or thoughts identify a realistic, actionable problem that you can solve in the near future? If so, they are productive. Listen long enough to understand what the underlying problem is, then quickly shift your focus to constructively solving the problem. If, on the other hand, the problem is beyond your control, those difficult emotions and thoughts are unproductive. Allow yourself to feel them from a distance then watch them fade away. If unproductive worries by definition have no rational answer, attempting to solve the unsolvable results in a never-ending circular pattern of thinking that quickly spins out of control.

Sometimes people get caught up in the search for perfect solutions. Note that you are looking for realistic, practical solutions—not perfection. If you are willing to only accept perfect solutions, you will refuse to take any possible risk. This fear of failure will also lock you into a similar recirculating cycle of worry and rumination.

It can be hard to think rationally, especially in moments of worry, fear or anger. In these moments, sometimes, all I can do is recite the famous Serenity Prayer:

"God, grant me the serenity to accept the things I cannot change, the courage to change the things that I can, and the wisdom to know the difference."[41]

If I persistently seek this truth, I reduce the urgency to make uncomfortable emotions and thoughts immediately disappear, I calm the difficult emotions in my body, and I wield the Sword of Truth. I eventually discover healthier paths for becoming a better version of myself.

6. Reassess their intensities

As you repetitively wield your new Sword of Truth, you will develop more rational counterarguments. These will become your new

---

41   Reinhold Neibuhr, Serenity Prayer (1892-1971)

automatic way of thinking, but it takes time. Remember the Colorado River. You are trying to gradually etch new, healthy, less-destructive thinking channels in your brain.

After using your Sword of Truth, reevaluate the intensity and validity of your difficult emotions and thoughts. Do they seem as severe now? Do they feel as true? Record the new intensity level on the scale from 0-100. Note how close you are to your goal. Remember we are not searching for perfection, just progress.

After working with this mood journaling process for a while, these patterns of attenuating your emotions and reassessing your thinking will become more automatic—as they did for one of my clients, Sharon. Sharon was sitting on the couch reading a book when her husband Greg walked into the house with his arms loaded with groceries. He snapped, "Well aren't you going to help me?" Sharon felt a flash of anger, and inwardly she thought, "What did I do? Why is he mad at me? Greg is a jerk!" Fortunately, she didn't convey these automatic thoughts.

She took a few deep breaths, slowed down her thinking processes and began to look for alternative explanations. She thought for a few seconds and even though they didn't feel absolutely true in the moment, she made a mental list of alternative explanations for his behavior:

1. Maybe he had a bad day at work.

2. Maybe he's worried about something: our finances, our son's grades, his mother's health, the election, the recent viral pandemic—God only knows life can be stressful.

3. Maybe somebody cut him off on the freeway. I know how aggressive drivers can make me angry.

4. Maybe he's hungry. I know how he gets "hangry" if he hasn't eaten in a while.

After identifying several alternatives, she decided that her immediate reaction was unproductive. She understood that part of Greg may be angry or frustrated, but she also knew that part of him loved her. She decided to use her Mountaintop Observer tool and just let the anger dissipate and flow away.

Ideally that's how things would work all the time, but we don't live in a perfect world. Especially in the beginning, your old automatic habits will kick in and you'll speak what's on your mind despite knowing it will escalate the problem. Later in the day, when you're calm and no longer emotionally flooded, pull out your Self-Care Journal and deliberately work through this encounter. Write down your immediate thoughts and reactions and then identify the components of the Sword of Truth that you think will help your situation. The more frequently you do this, the more quickly you will rewire your unhelpful, unhealthy automatic reactions.

The Emerald and the Crystal

When a friend of mine heard that my wife, daughter and I were traveling to the Grand Canyon, he recommended I read The Emerald Mile by Kevin Fedarko. I became so intrigued with the story that I researched all I could find about it, including archived interviews of Kenton Grua from Northern Arizona University, and There's This River: Grand Canyon Boatman Stories by Christa Sadler. This is a short synopsis of that material. If you like history, adventure and the outdoors, The Emerald Mile is a well-written, captivating narrative of Grua's life that I highly recommend you read.

Crystal Rapid has always been one of the most exciting series of rapids along the Colorado River. It uniquely rests at the merger of two canyons, Crystal Creek and Slate Creek. These canyons are steep, sparsely vegetated and filled with loose debris. When mixed with heavy rainfall, these three features can form large moving masses of loose sand, soil, rock, water, and air. These are not simply trickles of dirty water. They can develop into high-velocity rivers of undulating boulders, rocks and mud. In the case of Crystal Rapid, the two merging canyons deposit debris fans into the Colorado River from both sides at a single point, creating the unique and treacherous characteristics of its rapids. (Figure 4.4)

In 1966, fourteen inches of rain fell on the North Rim, producing a massive debris flow down Crystal Creek Canyon, altering Crystal Rapids in one of the largest geomorphic changes of the Colorado in recorded history. As it flowed into the Colorado it constricted the Grand Canyon to 25 percent of its previous width and deposited a large boulder at the top of the rapid, creating one of the largest and most dangerous hydraulics—or holes—on the river.

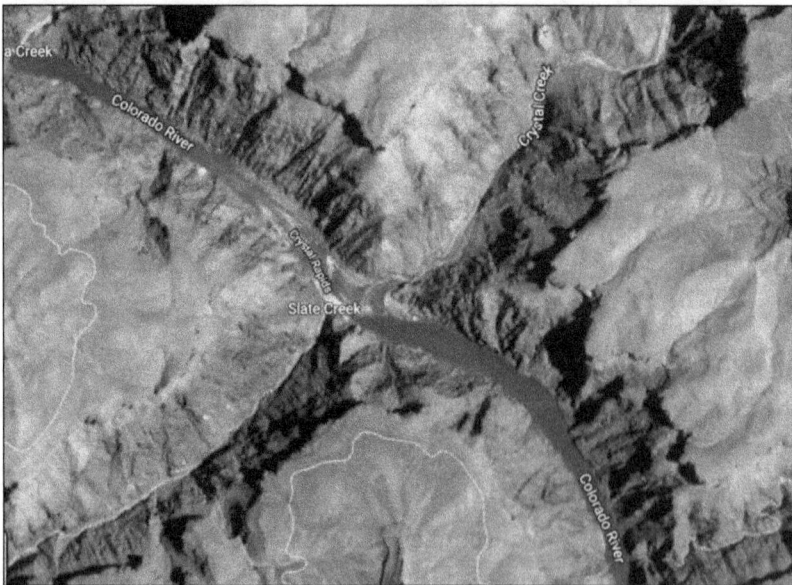

(FIGURE 4.4)

When water pours over the top of a submerged boulder or ledge, the current splits into two opposing streams. The surface water flows back upstream toward the object and the deep water continues to flow downstream. The result is a recirculating hole. Large objects of any kind, even boats, trees and people, can get trapped under the surface of these recirculating currents. When high flow rates collide with large obstacles, dangerous recirculating holes form what white-water enthusiasts refer to as "Keeper Holes." (Figure 4.5)

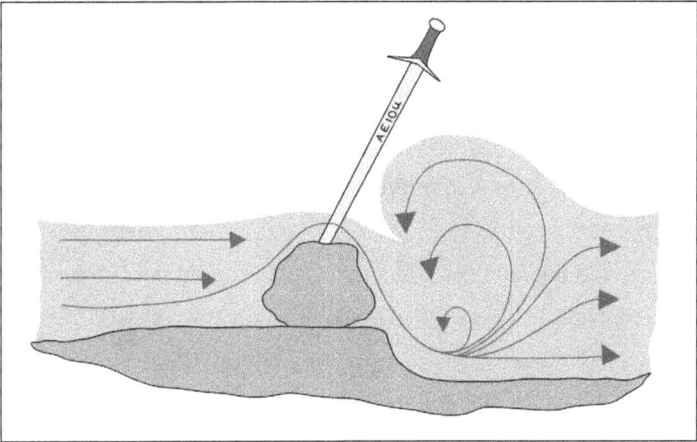

(FIGURE 4.5)

Note the similarity of how our own life storms can deposit sub-conscious, hidden obstacles that threaten to ensnare us in unhealthy recirculating thought patterns.

The storm of 1966 birthed a monster overnight. Crystal Rapid became one of the most feared and technical rapids in the Grand Canyon. Its boiling waters and gargantuan keeper hole have caused more boating accidents and deaths than any other single rapid on the river.

In the winter of 1982, the Pacific region experienced the worst El Niño in recorded history, unleashing a series of superstorms. To ease the increasing pressure on the Glen Canyon Dam, the Bureau of Reclamation diverted as much water through the hydroelectric turbines as possible, but Lake Powell continued to rise. The emergency spillway tunnels were opened to further divert water downstream, increasing the flow rate of the Colorado to over 70,000 cubic feet per second (cfs.)

When Lake Powell was initially filling, flow rates vacillated significantly. At night they dropped as low as 1,000 cfs, but during the day they increased as high as 28,000 cfs. To give you perspective, as I write this book in December of 2020, flow rates range from 9-16,000 cfs. According to Grua, "17,000-18,000 is pretty forgiving water."[42] At 70,000 cfs, nobody knew what to expect, and Crystal Rapid was taking on a new menacing form. At 70,000 cfs, the river—now traveling 30 mph—collided into a massive recirculating wall of water standing over thirty feet high.

During this harsh winter of 1982, Grua recognized the significance for the Colorado River and the possible conditions it would create for a record-setting river run through the canyon. Grua also understood that any mistake on the river now could be deadly, but the Canyon's tentacles tightly clutched him.

A few years earlier, Grua and two other boatmen set the current speed record through the Canyon, but now he had a chance to set one that would be impossible to beat, whether rowing or motoring. Grua was addicted. Escalating risk and achievement were his toxic drugs of choice.

At 11:00 p.m. on June 25, 1983, Grua and his two-man crew, Rudi Petschek and Steve "Wren" Reynolds, slipped Grua's little wooden boat, The Emerald Mile, into the tumultuous waters of Lee's Ferry. Grua knew their biggest challenge would come at mile ninety-eight, where Crystal was growing into an unfathomable beast. If they had any chance to survive her clutches, they must fight her during

---

42 Kevin Fedarko, *The Emerald Mile: The Epic Story of The Fastest Ride in History Through The Heart of The Grand Canyon* (Scribner, 2013).

daylight. This meant they must tackle the "less-threatening" initial sections under the veil of darkness.

As the sun began to peek over the rim of the canyon, Grua and his fellow oarsmen could hear Crystal, like the sirens of Odysseus, calling them in the distance. In an effort to save time, they decided not to stop and scout Crystal, choosing instead to row into the rapid blind.

Despite Grua rowing with all his might, Crystal grabbed The Emerald Mile and relentlessly pulled her in. Grua had no recourse but to point the bow directly into the three-story-tall wall of water. For a moment, he thought he saw a glimmer of hope through the center which might possibly save them. They braced as The Emerald Mile shuddered with the violent turbulence. The little dory continued to climb the massive wall, precariously balancing on her stern. Like a disrespectful suitor, Crystal slapped her one final time, flipping The Emerald Mile end over end and spinning her into the undertow. "The flip was instantaneous," said Petschek. "There was nothing rhythmic or graceful or easy about it at all. It was just—boom—we were over."[43]

Wren suffered the brunt of her anger. His account provides us with the richest details of what happened next, "That was the biggest wave I've ever seen. And he (Grua) hit it perfect. I don't think we could have hit it any better."[44] When the 1,100-pound boat slammed from its perch above, it slashed Wren's forehead and sent him deep into the bowels of Crystal. He remembers tumbling around as though he were in a washing machine for what seemed like an eternity. As Crystal pulled him deeper into her inner sanctum, he remembered being all alone as it grew darker and colder.

---

43 Chirsta Sadler, *There's this River: Grand Canyon Boatman Stories 2nd Edition* (This Earth Press, 2006).

44 Chirsta Sadler, *There's this River: Grand Canyon Boatman Stories 2nd Edition* (This Earth Press, 2006).

Prevailing wisdom teaches to curl into a ball and hope that you get caught in the downstream current at the bottom of the river. In theory, this will eventually take you to the surface, hopefully before you run out of breath and pass out. Wren, realizing this wasn't working, decided he needed to do something different or he was going to die. He began to swim with all his might, and then—inexplicably—Crystal released him. Twenty feet downstream, he found Grua and Petschek alive and attempting to right The Emerald Mile.

All three men relented to Crystal's recirculating currents, brushed her belly and accepted their fate. For reasons unknown, or maybe just sheer luck, they all emerged on the other side alive but changed, none more than Grua.

At 11:38 a.m. on June 27, Grua, Wren and Petschek entered the Lake Mead Reservoir, marking the end of their journey. Two hundred and seventy-seven miles from their starting point at Lee's Ferry, The Emerald Mile and her crew completed their quest in a record-breaking time of thirty-six hours, thirty-eight minutes, and twenty-nine seconds, shattering Grua's previous record by more than ten hours. To put that in perspective, most motorized rubber rafts complete the trek in about a week, and most wooden dories in two weeks.

At the age of fifty-two, while mountain biking on a beautiful day in the hills of Flagstaff, Arizona, Grua died of an aortic dissection. What the historic keeper hole of Crystal Rapids couldn't accomplish, an average mountain bike ride did. His life reminds us that our journey is fleeting, and that the end often comes without warning. It also reminds us that our best triumphs most often run through the heart of our desperate struggles if we are brave enough to face them.

The Canyon Rim and the River Below

While sitting on a rocky outcropping, with my feet dangling over the wall, I felt the Canyon's vastness and—in contrast—the smallness and temporal nature of my own life. I felt the primordial pull of the Canyon's beauty, yet simultaneously felt guilty for stepping away from my busy practice for the fourteen-day trip. My negative thoughts were pulling me into my own ruminating keeper hole of harsh self-criticism. My need to stay busy and prove my worth to myself and others by sacrificing my own mental health and relationships were automatic feelings that threatened to pull me under. I reminded myself that these thoughts were not necessarily all bad. At their core, they indicated that I cared, but I knew that unless I attenuated them they would grow to unhealthy levels.

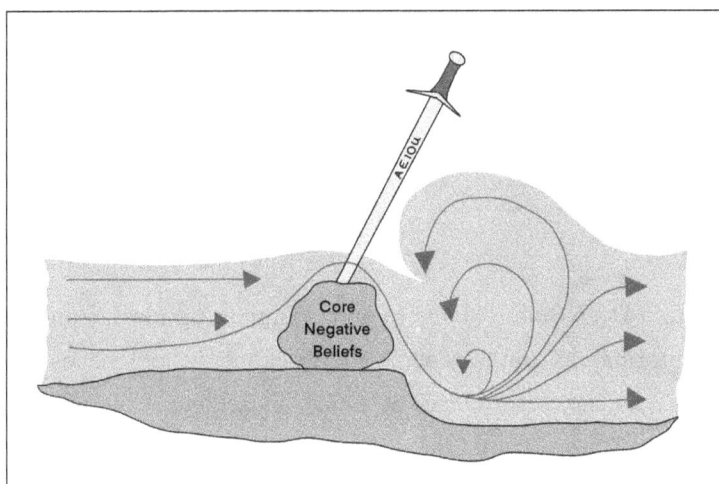

(FIGURE 4.6)

I decided to take a few breaths of the fresh, cool outdoor air and thrust a Sword of Truth into my recurrent voices of criticism. As I did, Grua's story percolated back into my thoughts, and I imagined seeing his little green dory, The Emerald Mile, floating down the river below. I continued to play with the image, visualizing those negative thoughts riding along on the dory's deck, not sinking them in the river or burying them in the sand. I allowed myself to feel the discomfort, to stay with them for the moment and evaluate their validity. I thought about my grandmother and what she would have said if she could hear me talk this way to myself.

With a little time and space, I began to recognize my cognitive distortions. As I did, the little dory eventually began to fade into the distance, and with it my recirculating harsh self-criticisms became less treacherous.

Life is short, as Grua's story reminds us, and like my trip to the Canyon, it will come to an end before we know it. In the end nobody remembers that I was absent from work those two weeks, and—truthfully—nobody cared. However, the three of us will remember those fourteen days for the rest of our lives. Attenuating my difficult emotions and thoughts helped shift my focus to the most important thing—my family—allowing me to stay present in the moment and enjoy our precious time together.

Summary

1. Your Deep Brain's ability to process almost limitless quantities of information simultaneously and at almost instantaneous speeds is amazing, yet it comes at a cost. To achieve these miraculous feats, it uses shortcuts to process information. These shortcuts, called heuristics, introduce errors. Sometimes the errors are not significant; other times they are quite problematic.

2. Psychologists call those shortcut-induced processing errors cognitive distortions.

3. With your Deep Brain handling the majority of the work in the background, your Surface Brain focuses on the single thing you deem important at the time.

4. Like difficult emotions, our natural desire is to destroy automatic negative thoughts (ANTs.) We want them to disappear.

But your ANTs contain information about your core values and represent at their most basic level something good about you. Obliterating them would destroy that information. A healthier approach to obliterating ANTs is to attenuate them or dial them down to more tolerable levels.

5. Writing is one of the most effective tools to help you process difficult feelings and dispute automatic negative thoughts and the cognitive distortions that feed them.

6. Mood Journaling is a practical writing tool that will help you process your difficult emotions and ANTs in more healthy ways.

The real hidden gem in the story of the Emerald and the Crystal is that none of us is immune to the recirculating undertows of automatic negative thoughts. Try as you may to steer clear of them, they have a tendency to pull you in. When they do, you have two choices:

1.) You can curl up in a ball at the bottom and passively submit. This is what most people do and as such they become consumed by their automatic negative thoughts.

Or:

2.) You can learn from Wren, who was swept into the bowels of Crystal. He decided that the conventional passive approach was not going to work and that if he didn't try something different, something unconventional, he was going to die. You too can choose a less common approach to contending with the undertows of automatic negative thoughts. Instead of yielding to the passive desire to obliterate your ANTs, decide to actively attenuate them. In the end, it is the Sword of Truth that will set you free.

Many people become imprisoned by their thoughts and emotions. Preserving the kernels of your ANTs that represent what is good and right about you is important because they provide you with something to expand upon and grow as you continue your journey of Empowered Self-Care. In the next chapter, **Assets**, we will plant those kernels and learn to cultivate them by focusing on the stories of your natural abilities and achievements.

CHAPTER 5

Assets — Discover Your Natural Gifts

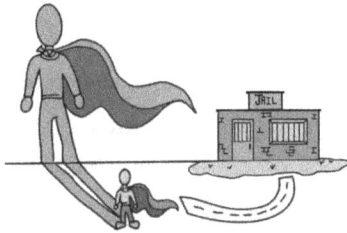

ARRIVAL GATE 1A: Adversity

DEPARTURE GATE 6A: Awareness, Attenuation, Assets, Allies, Aim, Action

Boarding Pass	Empowered Self-Care	Boarding Pass
Username: _____	**First Class**	← ✓ Departures
Destination: Beautiful Life	Current Location: Reality	✈ **6A**
Arrival: **Gate 1A** (Adversity)		Gate
Departure: **Gate 6A** (Awareness, Attenuation, Assets, Allies, Aim, Action)		

Most people think: success is achieved by correcting and fortifying their weaknesses.

The truth is: the most successful people capitalize on their inherent strengths.

"Everybody is a genius. But if you judge a fish by its ability to climb a tree, it will live its whole life believing that it is stupid."[45]

"Most people think they know what they are good at. They are usually wrong ... And yet, a person can perform only from strength."[46]

"What happens when we live God's way? He brings gifts into our lives, much the same way as fruit appears in an orchard—things like affection for others, exuberance for life and serenity. We develop a willingness to stick with things, a sense of compassion in the heart, and a conviction that a basic holiness permeates things and people. Since this is the kind of life we have (deliberately) chosen [...] let us make sure that we don't just hold it as an idea in our heads or a sentiment in our hearts, but work out (take action on) its implications in every detail of our lives ... that means we will not compare ourselves with each other [...] we have far more interesting things to do with our lives. Each of us is unique."[47]

G illian Pyrke grew up in the 1930s. She described herself as a reckless tomboy who climbed over boulders, ran through grassy meadows and explored pools of water with the boys who visited her family's cottage. Nowhere in her autobiography does she mention playing with dolls or sipping tea. She was always on the go, so much

---

45 Anonymous. This quote has historically been attributed to Albert Einstein; however, most believe that is not true, and nobody seems to agree who actually said it.

46 Peter Drucker, Alan Kantrow, Rick Wartzman and Julia Kirby, *Get the Right Things Done: The Drucker Collection* (Harvard Business Review Press, 2016).

47 Galatians 5:22-26.

so that her family said she "suffered from some kind of excess energy,"[48] nicknaming her "Wriggle-bottom."[49]

While excess energy might have seemed a nuisance for her parents, it caused even more problems when she started going to school. Her teachers thought she had a learning disability. While they attempted to lecture, Gillian couldn't keep quiet or still. She wanted to explore and play with the other children and was constantly disrupting class. Her teachers would place her back in her seat, but in a few minutes she was back up. Reprimands didn't settle her down either. Her entire life was one admonishment after another by some type of authority figure. At their wits' end, her teachers finally insisted her parents enroll her in a school for children with special needs.

Fortunately, her mother resisted. Even at a young age, Gillian understood the implications of going to a "special school." She didn't feel like there was anything wrong with her; her teachers just didn't understand her.

In The Element, Dr. Ken Robinson writes that Gillian's mother took her to a psychologist. In her autobiography, A Dancer in Wartime, however, Gillian says her mother took her to see their family's general practitioner. This is an important distinction that has implications for our healthcare system today. He knew her well. She had been "sickly," as she describes herself and as such had been a common fixture in his office.

She understood, however, that this visit was different from all her previous ones. Even with her childlike understanding, she knew it carried more importance. Gillian recalled some seventy years later that she felt nervous as she walked into his office filled with big oak

---

48   Gillian Lynne, *A Dancer in Wartime: The touching true story of a young girl's journey from the Blitz to the Bright Lights* (Vintage Books, Reprint edition, November 9, 2012).

49   Gillian Lynne, *A Dancer in Wartime: The touching true story of a young girl's journey from the Blitz to the Bright Lights* (Vintage Books, Reprint edition, November 9, 2012).

cabinets and leather chairs. Her mother passionately described her frustrations with Gillian's hyperactivity and her concerns that her teachers insisted they enroll her in a school for children with special needs. The wise physician listened intently, but more importantly he watched Gillian. He remembered all the other reasons for which Gillian had been in his office: the skinned knees, the cuts, the bruises. She was always getting into mischief.

He paused for a minute and asked Gillian's mother to step into the hall so they could speak in private, but before they left the room he walked over to the radio and turned it on. As they left, he turned to Gillian and sternly emphasized, "Young lady, you stay here."

Gillian's own words of the experience do it more justice than I can describe. "Out they went and the minute they had gone, I started to dance to the music, even going up on his desk because it seemed like a wonderful vantage point for jumping off from. What I hadn't noticed was that his door was one of those beautiful old glass ones with etched designs, through which the doctor and my mother were watching."[50]

The doctor looked at Mrs. Pyrke and told her, "She isn't sick. She's a dancer. Take her to dance school."[51]

If you don't recognize the name Gillian Pyrke, that is understandable. We know her now as Gillian Lynne. Gillian Lynne was one of Broadway's most prolific choreographers. She is best remembered for working on two of the longest running shows on Broadway, Cats and The Phantom of the Opera.

Gillian was fortunate. She had an established relationship with a general practitioner who was personally invested in her wellbeing. He was willing to take the time to listen and to watch. Gillian said,

---

50 Gillian Lynne, *A Dancer in Wartime: The touching true story of a young girl's journey from the Blitz to the Bright Lights* (Vintage Books, Reprint edition, November 9, 2012).

51 Ken Robinson, *The Element: How Finding Your Passion Changes Everything* (Penguin Books, 2009).

"Nowadays I dare say I would have been labelled with 'hyperactive'."
She's right. If she had gone to a busy primary care provider today,
the physician might have spent ten minutes with her, diagnosed her
with ADHD (Attention Deficit Hyperactivity Disorder) and given her
a prescription for Adderall or Ritalin.

What a tragedy it would have been if Gillian's mother had accepted
the education system's verdict or if her doctor had rushed in and
rushed out as so many physicians do today. We may have never experienced the gift of her unique work. The same applies to you. If you
fail to understand, use and advocate for your giftedness, you rob us of
your unique work.

Healing with Strength

In this chapter, I define **Assets** as the combination of your unique
strengths and the things you are naturally interested in doing. When
these two things collide, they produce your unique set of superpow-
ers. Through the recognition and development of these gifts you will
see the most success and meaning. You will discover later in this chapter how to recognize and interpret your behaviors to unlock your gifts.

Our school systems are good at training people en masse to work
in an industrialized economy. They are efficient at educating a population as a whole with a generalized approach; however, many people
finish school feeling inapt and defective. Our education system may
have been useful when our economy was based on factory work, but
now it is based on knowledge work.

Traditional education encourages rote memory. In our new knowl-
edge-work economy, people must be able to think for themselves.
They must be able to take disparate ideas and connect them in unique
ways. To stay competitive, companies are looking for individuals
who can view problems through different perspectives and generate creative solutions. People do this best when they understand and

utilize their unique giftedness. Our schools' current one-size-fits-all industrialized method does not appreciate peoples' unique gifts and learning styles.

Gillian's old physician was wise before his time. He slowed down and listened to Gillian's story. He watched her behavior. Your personal stories are your unique actions and behaviors, your innate choreographed dance. Your stories can be just as telling. Like Clayton Christensen, who employed the Jobs Theory by watching people's behaviors to discern why they were buying milkshakes, you can learn much about yourself from your own behaviors. You just need to know how.

The healing process should encompass mending the parts of us that are broken, but even more importantly it needs to emphasize all the parts that are healthy, all that is strong and all that is right about an individual.

In the 1960s, Martin Seligman threw the study of psychology into a tailspin. He insisted that we cannot heal people by simply removing disease. Picture a drowning person. If you pull him out of the depths of the sea, but leave him floating in the middle of the ocean, have you really saved him? No.

People want more than to just not drown. They want more than to be left floating in a sea of ambiguity and numbness. They want to soar.

I contend, like Seligman, that we want more than to merely survive. We want to thrive. We want to excel. We want our lives to count for something bigger than ourselves. We intrinsically thirst for meaning and fulfillment. I have discovered, as Dr. Christensen emphasized, your past and ongoing behaviors are the key to your thriving in the future.

In 2018, Martin Seligman and Tayyab Rashid wrote *Positive Psychotherapy: Clinical Manual*. It represents the culmination of Dr. Seligman's lifelong research in a single therapeutic system. The heart of his system focuses on what he calls "Character Strengths and

Signature Strengths." Once you have identified your unique strengths, he leads you through a journey of creating a better version of yourself and an action plan to implement that vision. Dr. Seligman says, "Assessing strengths along with symptoms is critical for a balanced and holistic clinical practice, and for understanding that psychotherapy is as much about cultivation of thriving as it is about alleviation of distress. Fixing weaknesses is remediation, whereas nurturing strengths produces growth and more wellbeing."[52]

Infectivity of Success

Recognizing and acknowledging your natural strengths can be a powerful way to motivate yourself to change. It instills confidence and helps you develop new personalized creative strategies to overcome obstacles. Just as thinking about problems can be contagious, thinking about your abilities can be too.

A simple way to begin the process of identifying your natural strengths is to read through a list of attributes or qualities of successful changers and see if any of those resonate with you. In Figure 5.1, you will find such a list created by W. R. Miller and Shelby Steen for behavioral intervention research. Circle all the strengths you think are applicable to you. List them in your journal.

Maybe you already know something about yourself that you don't see on this list. Record that in your journal. Think about a situation when you didn't believe you were going to succeed, but did. What ability did you draw upon to propel you forward? Spend some time writing about these. As you do, think about new situations in which you can use these strengths to succeed.

---

52 Tayyab Rashid and Martin Seligman, *Positive Psychotherapy: Clinician Manual* (Oxford University Press, 2018).

SOME CHARACTERISTICS OF SUCCESSFUL CHANGERS

Accepting	Committed	Flexible	Persevering	Stubborn
Active	Competent	Focused	Persistent	Thankful
Adaptable	Concerned	Forgiving	Positive	Thorough
Adventuresome	Confident	Forward-looking	Powerful	Thoughtful
Affectionate	Considerate	Free	Prayerful	Tough
Affirmative	Courageous	Happy	Quick	Trusting
Alert	Creative	Healthy	Reasonable	Trustworthy
Alive	Decisive	Hopeful	Receptive	Truthful
Ambitious	Dedicated	Imaginative	Relaxed	Understanding
Anchored	Determined	Ingenious	Reliable	Unique
Assertive	Die-hard	Intelligent	Resourceful	Unstoppable
Assured	Diligent	Knowledgeable	Responsible	Vigorous
Attentive	Doer	Loving	Sensible	Visionary
Bold	Eager	Mature	Skillful	Whole
Brave	Earnest	Open	Solid	Willing
Bright	Effective	Optimistic	Spiritual	Winning
Capable	Energetic	Orderly	Stable	Wise
Careful	Experienced	Organized	Steady	Worthy
Cheerful	Faithful	Patient	Straight	Zealous
Clever	Fearless	Perceptive	Strong	Zestful

"Some Characteristics of Successful Changers" is in the public domain and may be reproduced and adapted without further permission. This list, compiled by Shelby Steen, is from Miller, W.R. (Ed.). (2004). Combined behavioral intervention: A clinical research guide for therapists treating individuals with alcohol abuse and dependence (COMBINE Monograph Series, Vol. 1). Bethesda, MD: National Institute on Alcohol Abuse and Alcoholism.

(FIGURE 5.1)

How confident are you, on a scale of 0-10, that you can change and overcome an obstacle with which you are struggling? Why did you not choose some number lower than the one you selected? What would it take to move you up the scale to a higher number? Write your answers in your journal.

Popular Personality or Aptitude Tests

Sometimes your assets may be more difficult to recognize. What then? Over the years, many psychometric/personality/aptitude tools have been developed to help answer this question. I have taken several of these and have had my children take them as well. All have yielded helpful insights, but none seemed complete. I was looking for my personal owner's manual, something that would tell me how I work and what to do when I break myself. Have you ever wanted this?

Organizations ranging from the military to large corporations, academic centers and outpatient psychology clinics use versions of these tests. They are popular because they are simple to score and can easily be used to test large-scale populations. They are, however, subjective and dependent on the test taker's mood and desire to complete the test. They rely on a person's insight into their own abilities, and none of the tests consider a person's inherent motivation to use their aptitude.

My first encounter with aptitude testing came in the 1980s when, as a junior, my high school required us to take the Armed Services Vocational Aptitude Battery Test. It's a three-hour test that the Defense Department developed and uses to, "predict future academic and occupational success." The Defense Department promotes the test as a free service to help high school students determine career options in which they may be most successful. Obviously, it is used as a recruiting tool for the military and a mechanism for the Defense Department to assess the skills of the US student population.

I don't remember much about the test, but I do recall that it suggested my number one aptitude was nuclear physics. Not to deny the validity of the army's test, but I think they just had a shortage of physicists. Not long after taking the test, an army recruiter called, offering to pay for my education if I would study nuclear physics and commit to joining the army.

I saw three problems with this:

1. I didn't want to join the military.

2. While I liked the study of physics, I enjoyed working with people more. Locked in a gray office all day running equations and simulations on a computer seemed like torture.

3. Most importantly, I wanted no part of developing weapons of mass destruction.

I may have had an aptitude for something, but I had no motivation to do it. The army aptitude test did correctly identify an aptitude for visualizing theoretical concepts in concrete terms, but it could not identify my innate desire to do something. The test appeared to serve the Defense Department's needs more than it did mine. My first exposure to aptitude testing was a failure. I ignored it and went on to medical school. In retrospect, the main problem with the army's aptitude test was more than its failure to detect motivation. It was how the army insisted on using the information. It tried to assign me a specific job based on a single aptitude. Aptitudes don't tell you what to do exactly. They tell you how you naturally do things. After my first aptitude test, I was still looking for my personal owner's manual.

Five of the most popular psychometric tests used are the Big Five Model, DiSC, Myers-Briggs, StrengthsFinder and Enneagram. To give you an idea of the type of information they generate, I have listed a description of each, along with my results. I share my personal results simply as examples, not for comparison's sake. Each of our aptitudes and gifts is special and important. Consider doing one or more of these assessments yourself. None will paint the total picture of who you are, but each can help you discover unique aspects of your natural assets.

Our communities need the gamut of all our gifts. If you don't know and use your assets, our communities suffer. I hope that seeing my results will help you discover the distinctions between the various psychometric tools more clearly.

The Five Factor Model

The Five Factor Model is one of the newer versions, conceived in the 1980s. Since then, its structure continues to be refined and researched. It is based on the premise that we all exhibit aspects of five basic traits using the acronym **OCEAN:**

1. **Openness to Experience:** Openness (creativity and aesthetic sensitivity) and Intellect (interest in abstract concepts and ideas.)

2. **Conscientiousness:** Industriousness (the ability to engage in sustained, goal-directed effort) and Orderliness (the tendency to schedule, organize and systematize.)

3. **Extraversion:** Enthusiasm (spontaneous joy and engagement) and Assertiveness (social dominance, often verbal in nature.)

4. **Agreeableness:** Compassion (the tendency to empathically experience the emotion of others) and Politeness (the proclivity to abide by interpersonal norms.)

5. **Neuroticism:** Withdrawal (the tendency to avoid in the face of uncertainty) and Volatility (the tendency to become irritable and upset when things go wrong.)

Using a scale from "strongly agree" to "strongly disagree," the model asks you to answer 100 researched questions, which takes approximately fifteen minutes. The version I took was the Big Five Aspects Scale at www.understandmyself.com. With this particular version, your results for each of the five traits are compared in percentile form to over 10,000 other testees. Along with a comparative score, the test generates an eight-page descriptive report defining the traits and each of their two associated aspects, as well as the benefits and potential downsides of scores similar to yours.

My Score:

Openness (High experiences and ideas)

Conscientiousness (Moderately high industriousness and orderliness)

Extraversion (Low enthusiasm and average assertiveness)

Agreeableness (High compassion and politeness)

Neuroticism (Average withdrawal and volatility)

Myers-Briggs Type Indicator

The MBTI was originally developed by Katharine Cook Briggs and her daughter Isabel Briggs Myers as a tool to help women enter the workforce for the first time during WWII. Briggs began her research into personality around 1917, however it wasn't until 1944 when she and her daughter published their first MBTI handbook.

The premise of the MBTI is roughly based on Carl Jung's clinical observations that people experience the world using four psychological functions: **Sensation, Intuition, Feeling,** and **Thinking.**

MBTI defines four categories of opposing descriptors using Jung's personality terms:

- Extraversion/Introversion (E or I)
- Sensing/Intuition (S or N)
- Thinking/Feeling (T or F)
- Judging/Perceiving (J or P)

According to the MBTI philosophy, people naturally prefer one or the other in each pair, much like you prefer using either your right or left hand. As a result, sixteen possible personality types exist as a combination of these preferences.

Your MBTI type is reported as a four-letter sequence that represents your preference for each of the four pairs of descriptors.

One of the difficulties in understanding the MBTI is that it defines these descriptors differently from how they are used in everyday speech. The other difficulty is understanding how the four sets of descriptors relate to each other.

The two outer pairs, Extraversion/Introversion and Judging/Perceiving, are called attitudes and tell you how you interact with the world. The first pair, Extraversion/Introversion indicates what energizes you. The last pair, Judging/Perceiving points to the function you use predominantly.

The two middle pairs, Sensing/Intuition and Thinking/Feeling, are called your mental functions and tell you how your brain works. Sensing and Intuition are considered Perceiving functions, and Thinking and Feeling are considered Judging functions. Perceiving functions describe how we gather information, whereas Judging functions describe how we make decisions. You use all four of these mental functions, but prefer one from each pair. Let's break down each of the four pairs so you can start to make sense of the letters.

E/I: Extraversion or Introversion—How you are energized

- **Extraversion:** outwardly focused—draws energy from action—acts then reflect—seeks breadth of knowledge and influence—prefers more frequent interaction with people.

- **Introversion:** inwardly focused on a world of ideas and reflections—expends energy acting—builds energy through quiet time alone—reflects then acts—seeks depth of knowledge and influence—prefers fewer more substantive interactions with people.

S/N: Sensing or Intuition—How you gather information

- **Sensing:** (concrete thinker)—prefers concrete information gathered through the five senses—distrusts hunches—finds meaning directly in the data.

- **Intuiting:** (abstract thinker)—prefers concepts that link information in a wider context of patterns, theories and principles—discovers meaning in the broad metalaws that overlie and drive the data.

F/T: Feeling or Thinking—How you make decisions

- **Feeling:** (empathetic)—makes decisions by weighing perspectives to achieve a balance of greatest harmony/consensus/fit by considering people's needs.

- **Thinking:** (logical)—makes decisions from an emotionally detached perspective—prefers what makes sense logically, causally, consistent with known rules—has trouble interacting with people who don't think "logically"—tends to give very direct feedback—views truth as most important.

P/J: Perceiving or Judging—How your brain prefers to function

- **Perceiving:** prefers to gather information either through sensing or intuition.

- **Judging:** prefers to make decisions quickly and settle matters through either feeling or thinking.

As an example, the MBTI classifies me as an INFJ, but I think I am a blend of that and INTJ.

As an INFJ I am an introvert, which means I am energized by my world of ideas and reflections. I use feeling—or weighing perspectives—as my dominant inner function, and intuition—or conveying contextual patterns and theories—in my outer world. The MBTI website says that as an INFJ:

> "You seek meaning and connection in ideas, relationships, and even material possessions. You often want to understand what motivates others. You're conscientious and committed to your values and generally have a clear vision of how to best serve the common good. You're organized and decisive when trying to carry out your vision."[53]

Researchers question the statistical validity of the MBTI for several reasons.

1. Little evidence exists that people are dichotomous for each of the pairs. Most people lie somewhere in the middle, showing a mixture of each function.

2. The accuracy of the test, as with any questionnaire-based method, depends on honest self-reporting and a high level of personal awareness.

3. As we discussed earlier, the terminology is vague and inconsistent with the way these same terms are normally used.

4. The retest reliability is about 50 percent meaning that if you retake the test 5-6 weeks later, you likely fall into a different category.

---

53 The Myers-Briggs Company, https://explore.mbtionline.com/results.

Even with its limitations, I think the MBTI provides information that will help explain how you process information and relate to the world around you. At the same time, it can be difficult to understand. I would recommend you seek the aid of a good MBTI practitioner to help walk you through the process. Two Myers-Briggs websites (www.myersbriggs.org and www.themyersbriggs.com) are great online resources to help you test and understand your Myers-Briggs personality score. They also have links to consultants who can help explain your personality type if you need further information.

DiSC

DiSC is a more limited personality tool. Rather than describing a comprehensive personality type, it details how you approach making decisions and accomplishing tasks. It was originally developed in the 1920s by the psychologist, attorney, and writer William Marston. For all his groundbreaking work in psychology, Marston is best known for creating the cartoon character Wonder Woman, proving that we are all multifaceted individuals. His DiSC profile divides personalities into four basic domains: Dominance, Influence, Conscientiousness, and Steadiness.

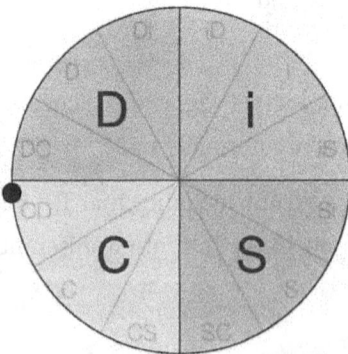

FIGURE 5.2

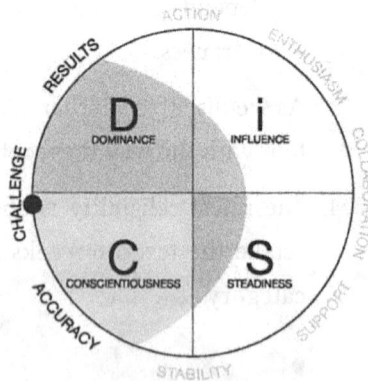

FIGURE 5.3

We are a combination of all four personalities, with some of us leaning more toward one type than another. Figures 5.2 and 5.3 are excerpts from my DiSC profile. The black dot represents my personality. Points on the perimeter suggest a strong correlation with a particular personality type and points closer to the center suggest less association.

People whose personality type falls dead center are an equal mix of all four. While my profile is a mix of Dominance and Conscientiousness, you can see in this graph how we are all a blend of the four personality types.

I scored as a "high CD," suggesting a strong correlation between conscientiousness and dominance. This correlates with the following characteristics:

- High expectations of myself and others

- Struggle to share responsibility with others

- Little patience for disorganized people

- Can be perceived as emotionally detached

- Stubbornness

- Pride myself in the quality of my work

- High problem-solving skills

- High determination

StrengthsFinder

In the late 1990s, Don Clifton assembled a team of scientists with the goal of developing a common language for talent. Their aim, as opposed to the common work of psychology that previously focused on what was wrong with people, was to create a system to help people understand what was right about themselves. They mined their database of 100,000 interviews and identified the thirty-four most common talent themes: achiever, activator, adaptability, analytical, arranger, belief, command, communication, competition, connectedness, consistency, context, deliberative, developer, discipline, empathy, focus, futuristic, harmony, ideation, includer, individualization, input, intellection, learner, maximizer, positivity, relator, responsibility, restorative, self-assurance, significance, strategic, and woo.

The Clifton StrengthsFinder assessment gives you twenty seconds to answer each of the 177 questions. Restricting the time forces you to give your initial automatic response, which the researchers felt better correlates with your true talents.

My results:

1. **Achiever:** Driven by the need to produce something tangible, relishes being busy, an internal fire pushes you to do more, must learn to cope with the constant feeling of discontent.

2. **Intellection:** Likes to think, enjoys time alone to muse and reflect, introspective, can lead to a sense of discontent as you compare what you are actually doing to all the ideas your mind conceives.

3. **Relator:** Take great pleasure in being around people you already know, comfortable in intimacy, relationships have value only if they are genuine.

4. **Futuristic:** You see in detail what the future might hold, this image pulls you into the future and inspires you to pursue it, people often find these visions inspiring, the future possibilities fascinate you.

5. **Learner:** Loves to learn, the process of learning is especially exciting more than the content or result, energized by the steady and deliberate journey from ignorance to competence, enticed

by the confidence of skills mastered, the outcome of learning is less significant than the "getting there."

Enneagram

The Enneagram is the oldest of the psychometric tests. Some say it may date back 3,500 years, but its age and etiology are widely disputed. "Ennea" is Greek for the number nine, and "gram" is Greek for "a drawing."

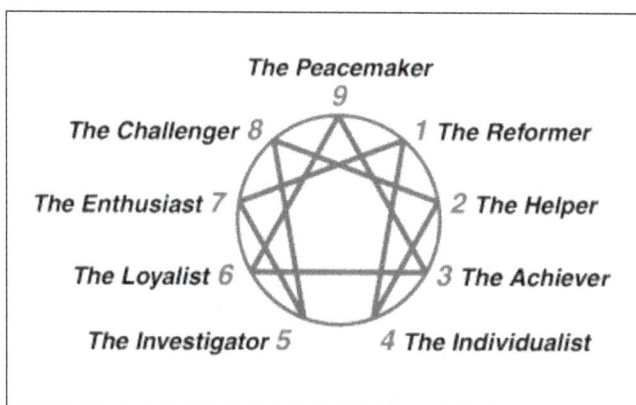

The Peacemaker
9
The Challenger 8   1 The Reformer
The Enthusiast 7   2 The Helper
The Loyalist 6   3 The Achiever
The Investigator 5   4 The Individualist

(FIGURE 5.4)

It is often depicted as a nine-sided polygon connecting nine central personal types. Unlike the other four personality tools, determining your personality or personhood through the Enneagram is more subjective. Modern experts have tried to simplify the process by developing checklists or questionnaires to aid in the process. I found determining my aptitudes or personality type with the Enneagram the most challenging. Each type has its own strengths and weaknesses, and behaviors can manifest differently depending on whether a person is healthy or unhealthy.

I used one of the several checklists available which suggested that I am an Enneagram 1 which some call The Reformer or The Perfectionist. The Investigator, Enneagram 5, was a close second. Truthfully, I recognize much of myself in both of those types.

Another resource I read discouraged using checklists and questionnaires. It suggested that you should look back into your teens and twenties, before you started your vocation, and explore why you did certain things. "Think more about how you act at home rather than work." The author encourages you to ignore your behaviors, saying, "Your number is not determined by what you do so much as *why* you do it."[54]

In the end, I settled on Enneagram 1 as my primary type: ethical, productive, idealistic, self-disciplined, fair, but can be critical (especially self-critical), obsessive-compulsive, and dissatisfied. Type 1s tend to compulsively worry about mistakes, fear failure and can be uncomfortable asking for their needs. Healthy 1s are committed to a life of service and integrity and are able to forgive themselves and others for being imperfect.

Enneagram 5 also feels natural to me: analytical, objective, self-contained. They love developing a thorough understanding of topics, but can be slow to apply that knowledge in the real world. As introverts, social settings typically drain them of energy. Healthy 5s maintain a good balance between observing and participating. They develop a depth of knowledge in several areas and are willing to share it with others.

If you are interested in learning more about the Enneagram, I recommend reading The Road Back to You by Ian Morgan Cron and Suzanne Stabile, and The Enneagram Made Easy by Renee Baron and Elizabeth Wagele.

---

54 Ian Morgan Cron and Suzanne Stabile, *The Road Back To You: An Enneagram Journey to Self Discovery* (InterVarsity Press, 2016).

There is no one perfect way to understand your natural assets. We are complex individuals with many nuances. Each of these tests has helped me understand my traits in a little different and meaningful way. It was once explained to me that personality testing is like a kaleidoscope. By looking at all of them you can see a fuller, more beautiful picture of yourself. At the same time, they can be confusing, and sometimes they look like a bunch of random shapes and colors.

While all five of these tools are helpful, they depend on similar questionnaires and test formats. The only exception is the Enneagram, about which some debate exists over the best way to implement the test. Questionnaires, by their very nature, glean insight by how you consciously answer a list of predetermined questions. You can only answer based on what you understand.

As Clayton Christensen suggested, sometimes we act for reasons we don't fully understand. We buy milkshakes in part because we like the way they taste, but maybe we also buy them because we are looking for an easy-to-consume, non-messy meal that keeps us satisfied all morning. The search for your assets is not dissimilar. This includes how you use your natural assets. You often use them subconsciously, and therefore may not recognize them. Another way to discover something about your innate strengths or assets is to study how you have naturally acted throughout your life.

The Story of Your Assets

Watching your behavior in the moment and understanding why you do something is difficult. Watching yourself retrospectively using story is easier. As I discussed in the introduction, story is the primary tool humans use to understand their situations and surrounding environments.

If we understand our behaviors and those of others through story, then why have psychometric and personality tests not incorporated it in their processes? One reason is that storytelling is slower and more nuanced; it's less scalable than computer-generated questionnaires. A narrative process takes time and the willingness to invest in others.

Unfortunately, in medicine the art of history taking and physical exams are dying. Modern physicians like to run tests. They're efficient. They don't require much time and they give clear, unambiguous answers. I am as guilty as any physician. Gathering a comprehensive medical history—a person's story—is more complex and nuanced. Psychology is no different. Instead of listening and watching, psychologists often use a number of psychometric tests to classify people's personalities. Tests simplify people into clear categories which makes them easier to understand. In these simplified versions of ourselves however, we sometimes miss uniqueness and nuance. That is not to say that standardized tests are unhelpful. As I have shown, they can be extremely useful, but I believe they are best used in combination with an individual's story.

In addition, healthcare providers are bad about attaching labels to people, though we prefer to use the term "diagnosis." We inadvertently pathologize behaviors that seem to fall outside the standard bell-shaped curve of normalcy. Unfortunately, these labels sometimes leave people feeling broken. They focus on all that seems wrong with an individual.

In the previous chapter, we discussed how it is easy to focus on all that is wrong with us, constraining and imprisoning ourselves in recirculating patterns of negative thoughts and behaviors. We learned, however, that our difficult emotions and negative thoughts are not all "bad." They also contain information that points to what is good and right about us. Contrary to typical methods of healing, self-help and correction, Empowered Self-Care focuses on healing with your own natural assets, all that is good and right about you.

Giftedness

The quest for understanding the story of your assets, or what we will refer to as the Giftedness Process, begins in the 1940s with Bernard Haldane. He initially trained as a physician in England, but discovered when he moved to New York in 1946 that his medical certification did not meet US standards. Searching for a different way to constructively serve people, Haldane noted that many young men who returned home at the end of WWII struggled to find a good fit in the job market. He postulated that age, education and experience were not barriers to success, but knowledge of someone's own values and strengths. He believed that people are often taught at home, in school and in many religious institutions attitudes and beliefs that limit their progress. These types of limitations are even noted in our children's stories. Take this passage from Alice's Adventures in Wonderland as an example:

> *"Alice:* Where I come from, people study what they are not good at in order to be able to do what they are good at. [...] Grown-ups tell us to find out what we did wrong, and never do it again.

> *Mad Hatter:* That's odd! It seems to me that in order to find out about something, you have to study it. And when you study it, you should become better at it. Why should you want to become better at something, and then never do it again? But please continue.

> *Alice:* Nobody ever tells us to study the right things we do. We're only supposed to learn from the wrong things. But we are permitted to study the right things other people do. And sometimes we're even told to copy them.

> *Mad Hatter:* That's cheating!

> *Alice:* You're quite right, Mr. Hatter. I do live in a topsy-turvy world. It seems like I have to do something wrong first, in order

to learn from that what not to do. And then, by not doing what I'm supposed to do, perhaps I'll be right. But I'd rather be right the first time, wouldn't you?"[55]

To help his clients discover their latent or unrealized strengths, Haldane asked people to write about ten experiences where they had accomplished something positive. He encouraged them to discard modesty and to record as many details as they could remember. He defined accomplishments as activities they enjoyed doing, did well, made them feel good when it was done, and brought them personal satisfaction. It didn't matter whether anybody else thought they were good at these activities. The only thing that mattered was what they thought about the activity at the time.

For example, an activity I wrote about was performing at family gatherings. I pretended to be Elvis, singing, playing my guitar and shaking my leg. In the grand view of history this is insignificant, but in the eyes of my six-year-old self, this was important. It brought my six-year-old self enjoyment and satisfaction, and I felt like I was good at it.

Achievement = activities you enjoyed doing, did well in your own eyes and that brought you satisfaction.

Once his clients completed their achievement stories, Haldane had them choose characteristics about themselves from a list of fifty-two traits of successful people—what he called "success factors"—that they could identify in each of their stories. This helped them recognize patterns in their diverse and often seemingly dissimilar achievements. As they identified their own success characteristics, they were to place a checkmark next to it on a chart. After completing this process for each of their ten stories, Haldane's clients were asked to tally the

---

55 Lewis Carroll, *Alice's Adventures in Wonderland* (1865).

DR. YOU

total number of checkmarks identified for each characteristic. Of the fifty-two, Haldane found that usually 8-10 characteristics had multiple checkmarks, and within this group typically only a few registered four checkmarks or more. These characteristics with four or more checkmarks defined what he called the client's Success Pattern. These are the success factors that contributed more to their achievements, enjoyment and satisfaction in the past and could be used to do the same in the future.

Next, he asked his clients to review their achievements and all their listed success factors and identify the ones they felt were subjectively the most important or aligned most with their core values. They were asked to go back and place a double check by these ones, then retally the list.

He cautioned his clients that as they did this to be aware of negative beliefs that may keep them from being honest with themselves.

All the success factors in their pattern were important, but especially those they deemed most significant and aligned with their most cherished values. These factors now became the core of Haldane's success exercise program. By devoting yourself to the maximal development of these factors, you develop long-term habits for success.

In an article titled *Bernard Haldane Was Ahead of His Time*, Jerald Forster wrote, "Bernard Haldane deserves the title of 'pioneer' in the optimization of behavior and the application of positive psychology [...] Bernard started to articulate methods of optimization in the 1950s and he continued to develop these methods into the 1990s [...] However, it was not until the 1990s that the theories and rationales for positive psychology and optimization through wellness became key concepts in the literature of psychology and counseling." Forster went on to say, "While the first part of Bernard's career was almost totally focused on the goal of facilitating job and career satisfaction, the latter part had a broader focus on what might be called life satisfaction."[56]

In 1958, Arthur Miller Jr., an attorney who had been promoted to head the personnel department of his company, invited Haldane to speak at a self-development seminar sponsored by the American Management Association. The session Haldane led was titled, *Building Resumes on the Basis of Successes One Has Experienced.* Miller says in his book, *The Power of Uniqueness: How to Become Who You Really Are,* "What he said about focusing on positive past experiences brought together a number of latent observations I had made over the years about the way people are put together [...] The paradigm I suddenly saw come together focused on the uniqueness of an individual—not on general principles or traits (like other available psychometric tests.)"[57]

For the next several decades, Miller devoted his life to researching and developing his own system for helping people discover their unique motivated abilities. His System for Identifying Motivated Abilities, like Haldane's, uses stories of individuals' past positive activities. He later founded a company bearing the same name as his system, SIMA, to promote his work. This system is a complex proprietary program that generates a 40+ page document explaining someone's giftedness.

The Soothsayer

About a year into my new practice, I met three people who over a span of three weeks all independently suggested that I meet Bill Hendricks. All three men were interested in my new model of

---

56 Jerald Forster, Professor Emeritus, College of Education, University of Washington, Bernard Haldane Was Ahead of His Time, https://www.thepositiveencourager.global/bernard-haldanes-approach-to-doing-positive-work/.

57 Arthur F. Miller, Jr. and William Hendricks, *The Power of Uniqueness: How to Become Who You Really Are* (Zondervan, 1999).

healthcare and wanted to help me build and promote my practice. One was a banker, one a philanthropist and the other a retired TV cable businessman. None of them were medical professionals, but all three were astute businessmen.

They described Bill as a soothsayer, a man who had an uncanny ability to discern a person's inner motivations and unique gifts. Intrigued, I grabbed a copy of his book, *The Person Called You: Why You're Here, Why You Matter & What You Should Do with Your Life*. I highly recommend that you read it. He also recently completed a second book with his sister, *So How Do I Parent This Child?: Discovering the Wisdom and the Wonder of Who Your Child Was Meant to Be*. It outlines a great way to help your child discover who they are intended to be.

As a young man struggling to find direction, Bill was encouraged by an acquaintance of his father to go through Art Miller's SIMA program. A talented wordsmith, Bill obtained a Bachelor of Arts degree in English from Harvard, a Masters in communications from Boston University, and a Masters in theology from Dallas Theological Seminary. As such, he was already primed for the critical discipline of parsing the hidden meaning in nuanced patterns of people's stories. This was a task he felt he was uniquely created to do. He was so impressed with the process that he immediately knew this was his life's work. Bill underwent the certification process and in 1985 opened his own consultant practice, The Giftedness Center, located in Dallas, Texas.

When I first met Bill, I felt I had discovered a long-lost kindred spirit. He walked me through the SIMA program, and I immediately recognized its potential in healthcare. As I have mentioned before, most of the time when people walk into my clinic with a chronic medical condition, they know what they need to do but lack the confidence and often the motivation to do it. As recent psychological studies have discovered, recognizing and understanding our innate strengths is an important component of boosting both confidence and motivation.

It is my belief, like Bill, that everybody is gifted with a unique set of strengths and interests because we are created to serve a unique purpose. Giftedness, as Bill explains it, is not about something that you can do, but something that you cannot not do. It is about something you are born to do and enjoy doing well. It is a process of becoming more of what is good and right about yourself.

Bill's words rang true to me and seemed consistent with what Dr. Seligman had discovered. They also reminded me of the concept of "flow" as described by psychologist and researcher Mihaly Csikszentmihalyi. Flow is the optimal life experience that occurs when we balance our skill set with the challenges we encounter. Csikszentmihalyi describes flow as, "The state in which people are so involved in an activity that nothing else seems to matter; the experience itself is so enjoyable that people will do it even at great cost, for the sheer sake of doing it."[58] In my experience, people encounter their most accelerated growth in this natural flow state.

In Figure 5.5, I have replaced the concept of flow with growth and skill set with the six tools I cover in this book. It illustrates how when Adversity exceeds our toolset, we become overwhelmed. When our skills significantly exceed our current challenge, we stagnate. We experience a state of growth when our challenge slightly exceeds our skills and encourages us to push beyond our present capacity.

This is the path that leads to meaning and fulfillment, or what I refer to as a "beautiful life." This path of meaning infuses the more menial tasks of life with purpose, as they become steps in the process of moving you toward something greater.

Note that simply possessing all the necessary tools does not yield growth. Beautiful living is the by-product of applying your tools, especially your natural Assets, to life's challenges. Without the

---

58 Mihaly Csikszentmihalyi, *Flow: The Psychology of Optimal Experience*, (Harper Perennial, 1991).

appropriate tools, we become overwhelmed, but also note that it is important to challenge ourselves. When we isolate ourselves from the outside world, from challenges, from differing opinions and points of view, and when we demand the protection of safe spaces, we stagnate. Just like muscles that atrophy when they are not exercised, we become emotionally weaker or, even worse, morose, depressed and unfulfilled. The path to beautiful living thus runs through the heart of adversity. As we acquire more tools and learn to use them more efficiently, we become stronger and more resilient to even greater levels of adversity.

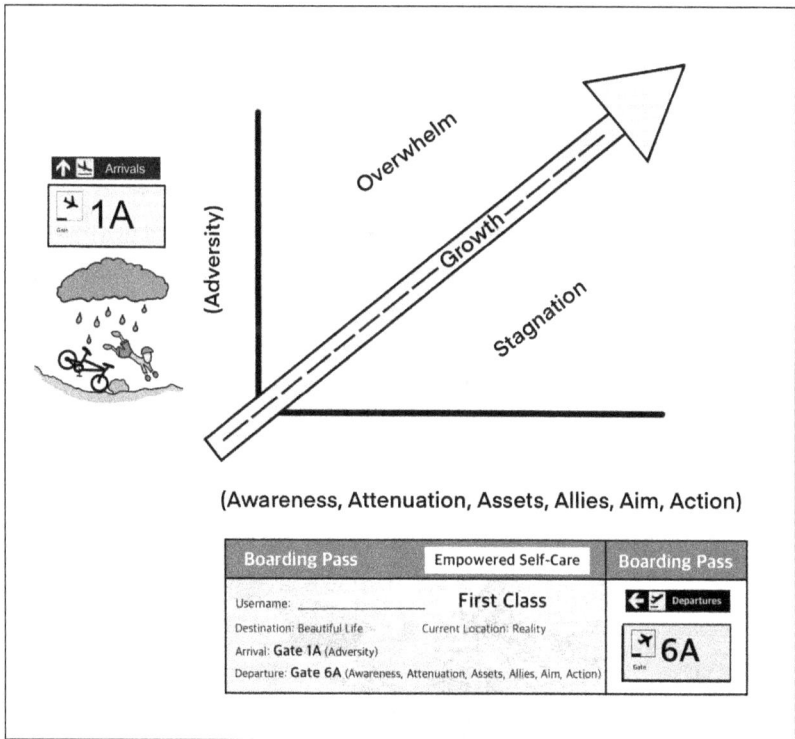

(FIGURE 5.5)

Another lesson to learn from this graph, specifically about your natural assets, is that you will become overwhelmed when you expect yourself to do things in areas you are not gifted. I don't care how much I practice shooting basketball, I will never be able to compete in the NBA. I can get better at shooting free throws, but if you threw me into an NBA game, it would be ugly. I would get massacred. I would feel completely overwhelmed and outclassed. It has been said, "If you judge a fish by its ability to climb a tree it will live its whole life believing that it is stupid."[59]

Some of what we consider to be depression, melancholy, hyperactivity or anxiety is at least in part due to people's inability to recognize and use their innate strengths and assets. They are trying to fit themselves into the world's puzzle like a round peg in a square hole. Like Gillian Lynne, there's nothing wrong with them, they are just trying to be something they were never intended to be.

Why is it so hard to clearly recognize our assets? We don't see our combination of skills and motivations as unique. We have always seen the world through our own perspective. We've never experienced the world any differently. We assume that everybody sees the world the same way. They don't.

Occasionally I lose my stethoscope—okay, frequently I lose my stethoscope. Rummaging around in the exam room while apologizing, I'll explain to my patients that I have the gift of losing things. To my embarrassment, they often point out that my stethoscope is hanging around my neck. Because it is always around my neck, I forget about it. Maybe you have experienced the same thing with your glasses. Your assets and giftedness are a little like that. They are always with us and have always been with us, so we often don't remember they are there.

---

59 Anonymous. This quote has historically been attributed to Albert Einstein; however, most believe that is not true, and nobody seems to agree who actually said it.

To help people learn how to identify their assets, I've adopted a simplified five-step giftedness process from Bill Hendricks that I use in my practice.

Five Steps to Discovering Your Giftedness:

1. List your stories.

2. Write or tell your stories.

3. Analyze your stories.

4. Look for the patterns.

5. Consolidate into a single statement.

Step 1: List Your Stories

Your Giftedness has been with you your entire life. It began manifesting when you were very young. Starting back as far as you can remember, look for stories of activities in which you lost yourself in the moment. These activities are ones that you found intrinsically motivating, meaning you did them naturally. You enjoyed them and were energized by them. You did these activities automatically with no encouragement from others. They may have praised you for doing them, but that was not your underlying motivation. You would have done them anyway. External validation of ability is of little importance in this discussion.

Whether or not you are better than other people with the same gift is not important. How skillful you are at a task depends not only on natural aptitude, but on the time you have spent developing your gift. Let's use the gift of drawing as an example. You may possess an aptitude for drawing, but have never spent time developing your technique. You are now fifty and your skill level has remained unchanged since the age of ten. You possess that raw gift, but compared to people who have spent the last forty years developing their craft, your gift doesn't seem to compare. Looking back, however, you remember that drawing was an activity in which you would completely lose yourself. You intrinsically felt you were good at it and—more importantly—derived much satisfaction from it. That is still an aptitude.

Now that you know what you are looking for, take an hour or so and write down the basic content of 10-15 such stories. Ideally, you want to include stories from each period of your life, starting back as far as you can remember.

Story Criteria Summary:

- Stories of activities. These are stories of things you actively performed, not something in which you passively participated.

- These activities should be something you intrinsically enjoyed and found satisfying.

Examples:

The following examples are compiled from several people I know, except the first, which you'll recognize as my own.

- Age eight: I sang in our family's annual Christmas talent show. Even then, I was a natural entertainer, shaking my leg, playing guitar and pretending to be Elvis.

- Age ten: Some people thought I was crazy. They would laugh at me when I told them I wanted to be an accountant. I helped my neighbors set up a budget and straighten their finances.

- Age twelve: I would draw and paint all day in my room. I would get so lost in what I was doing that my mother would have to come in and remind me to eat.

- Age thirteen: I loved to read and learn about anything and everything. Even when I was little, I found the Encyclopedia Britannica fascinating.

- Age sixteen: I volunteered every year at my local children's summer camp. I loved working with kids and seeing them grow.

- Age twenty: I opened and ran a specialty store selling old records along the main drag strip of my college campus.

- Age thirty-five: I set up a dedicated room in our house for quilting. I love stitching together different types of cloth with different colors and patterns to create a new single theme for the quilt.

- Age fifty-five: Nobody knows it, but I have been secretly writing poems for the last fifteen years. I find solace and peace in writing.

Reminder: When you think of your stories, keep these guides in mind:

A. Activities not experiences

Not: "I watched the sun rise on a mountaintop and felt closer to God and nature than ever before while I hiked a section of the Appalachian Trail."

But: "I had always dreamed of doing a thru-hike of the Appalachian Trail. I remember hiking a section of it in the Smoky Mountains when I was eight with my parents and thinking, 'Someday I am going to hike the entire AT.' When I was twenty-six, I found myself between jobs with nothing to prevent me from my dream hike. I spent three months researching shoes, backpacks, stoves, sleep systems, tents, and clothing options. I kept running lists of pros and cons of each article, including the size and weight of all my gear options. I watched every video and read every book I could find on hiking the AT. This past May, I started my trek and finished about six months later. What a wonderful adventure. I met so many fascinating, eccentric people, was able to submerge myself in a much more simplistic way of living, proved to myself that I could overcome countless obstacles, and gained a better perspective of my place in the world and the importance of the people in my life."

B. Activities not milestones

Not: "I completed my Master's degree in special education."

But: "After working with special needs children when I was on a high school mission trip to the Dominican Republic, I decided special education was my calling. As soon as I returned home, I called a grade school teacher who has acted as a mentor to me. She suggested an educational path that would help me achieve that goal. After a rocky start at one college, I transferred to another school that had a stronger education program. During school I worked in a local special education program as a teacher assistant. Juggling work and school was difficult, but I graduated with honors and was accepted into an online masters program. While working as a teacher assistant, I noticed that several of the children in the special ed program were also deaf and that few of the teachers could sign. Seeing a need, I simultaneously enrolled in a sign language certification program."

C. Give specific, detailed examples, not generalities

Not: "I like painting."

But: "When I was in the first grade, I got so excited when Mrs. Gordon told us we were going to have an art contest. All of the other children were making simple black-and-white drawings with their school pencils. I wanted my picture to burst with color and textures. I asked Mrs. Gordon to help me mix tempera paint, and painted an underwater world of sea creatures. I then cut out pieces of rubber, plastic, cloth, and cardboard in the shape of some of the images and glued them onto my painting. My underwater sea world came to life in 3D."

Now it's your turn!

Use the Story Highlights Form (Table 5.6) to help you organize and list your stories. Write just a sentence or two here, but be prepared to either tell or write each story in rich detail later. You can go to www.DrYou.org/resources to download a copy of the Story Highlight Form if you wish.

Step 2: Write or Tell Your Stories

Now that you have identified and written a basic description of 10-15 stories, if you feel comfortable, seek the help of a friend or acquaintance who is good at listening. You don't want somebody who will interrupt you or try to fix your perceived problems. Family members are usually too biased, so they don't typically make good listeners.

If you don't have anybody who can help, or you're not ready to involve another person, you can accomplish a similar function by writing your stories in detail. Write each story on a separate sheet of paper and make sure you cover all five elements of a successful story: Activity/Action, Subjects, Circumstances, Role, and Purpose/Satisfaction.

THE STORIES OF YOU

Age	Story Highlights

(FIGURE 5.6)

If you have chosen to tell your stories to a friend, set aside about an hour and a half to do so. You don't want to feel rushed. Pick a setting that is comfortable, quiet and has adequate privacy. Pull out your list and select your top eight stories. Close your eyes if you need to, and tell your stories as if describing a movie scene. Start with background information to give each story context. Describe the setting, where you were, who was with you, what you were doing, what were the circumstances surrounding the activity, and how you were doing it. Describe as many vivid details as possible. Make sure you include what you found satisfying about this activity. It should take you 10-15 minutes to tell each story in detail. Less than ten minutes and you probably didn't give enough detail, and more than fifteen minutes means you probably included too many extraneous details.

When I do this with patients and clients, I record the interview. This helps me focus on what they are saying without worrying that I may miss an important detail. I'd encourage you to do the same. As I listen, I ask clarifying questions to make sure they provide information about all five key elements of story: Activity, Subject Matter, Circumstances, Role, and Satisfaction. While I do take a few notes during the interview, I take most of them later when I am analyzing the recording.

Step 3: Analyze Your Stories

The recording allows both you and your friend to analyze your stories. I do this with my patients and clients first independently over about a two-week period, then we meet for an hour or two to discuss our findings.

As you review your recording, listen for specific words or phrases you used to describe the five key elements of story, then record those on individual Story Note forms.

1. **Abilities?** Look for action words (verbs) that describe the ability you use in the story.

2. **Subject Matter?** What things or people were you working on, with or through?

3. **Circumstances?** Circumstances are about the environment you were in. Was there stress and pressure? Were things calm and quiet? Were there a lot of people involved or just you? Were you working toward a goal or was your work flexible and unstructured? Was there a deadline? Was there an audience watching you? Were you being recognized or were you working behind the scenes? Were you outdoors or working inside? Where did your story take place? What were the conditions that affected how you did your activity? What factors motivated you to take action? What factors helped you sustain that motivation? Was there a structure that you preferred? What results were you trying to achieve?

4. **Role?** Were you a participant on a team? The leader? Did you organize everything? Did you function more like a teacher, coach or mentor? Did you function more as an individualist?

5. **Purpose/Satisfaction?** What were you trying to accomplish? What did you find so enjoyable or satisfying? What was the driving force that led you to participate in this activity?

STORY NOTES

Story:	
Abilities: *action words, verbs*	
Subject Matter: *objects of people that* *you worked on, with,* *or through*	
Circumstances: *setting, environment,* *conditions, triggers,* *motivations*	
Role: *how you interacted or* *related to others*	
Satisfaction: *what you found satisfying* *about the activity*	

(FIGURE 5.7)

Use the Story Note Template (Figure 5.7) to help organize your notes according to story. You can download copies at www.DrYou.org/resources.

After you both finish reviewing all your stories, take a break. I find it helpful to clear my mind and come back to the process with a fresh perspective.

Step 4: Look for Patterns

Using all your individual Story Note pages, look for patterns that connect the themes of your activity stories. For each of the five story elements, look for words or phrases that repeat themselves. They don't need to appear in all your stories, but you know they are important if you see them recur in four or five. Record these words or phrases on the Story Pattern form. Find all the patterns for each of the five elements that run through your stories.

Step 5: Consolidate into a Single Giftedness Statement

Write one or two sentences that summarize what you have discovered about yourself.

Melinda's Giftedness

For brevity's sake, I have presented only a small portion of Melinda's two-hour interview and have applied the giftedness process below only to the stories I have shared in this book. Hopefully this will give you a sample of what the full process looks like.

STORY PATTERNS

Abilities: *action words, verbs*	
Subject Matter: *objects of people that y ou worked on, with, or through*	
Circumstances: *setting, environment, conditions, triggers, motivations*	
Role: *how you interacted or related to others*	
Satisfaction: *what you found satisfying about the activity*	

(FIGURE 5.8)

Melinda struggled with depression for years. Like all the stories in this book, I have changed her name and some of the details of her story to protect her identity, but this story is consistent with the true underlying theme of our conversation.

Out of college Melinda started her own successful marketing company, but decided when she got married that it was time to devote herself to raising her family. Her husband was a successful executive, so her life of comfort continued until his company decided to restructure. Unemployed and in his mid-60s, he was competing with energetic younger candidates. These candidates had less experience, but companies could and did hire them at cheaper salaries. Nobody would directly admit it, but he was too old and overqualified.

After a couple of years of searching for a new managerial job, her husband finally gave up and started delivering pizzas and doing various minimum wage jobs. The family's savings subsequently dwindled to a critical low. Up until this point, Melinda had lived her entire life as part of the upper-middle class. She had always not only been financially secure, but she'd had more than she needed. Now she was about to lose her house. In her late fifties, Melinda decided to re-enter the workforce as an administrative assistant for a nonprofit organization just to pay the bills.

Melinda appreciated the mission statement of her employer, but the culture behind the good work was toxic and chaotic. She was already stressed with her family's financial problems and her husband's increasing depression, and now she was overwhelmed with the lack of structure and accountability in her new job. She was the primary administrative assistant for the CEO of the company and as such had an assistant of her own. Her assistant, however, was little help. She was in her late eighties and had been with the company since the beginning. As technology developed, her assistant didn't acquire any basic computer skills, much less the plethora needed to run a modern business office including its marketing and social media departments. To make matters worse, her assistant had memory problems, but because she had been with the company since the beginning the CEO would not replace her.

Melinda felt stuck. The job was killing her, but she needed the money. She was afraid to look for another. Her family was in no financial position to take any more risks. She wanted to start her own business, but that wasn't an option. Melinda's depression began to spiral out of control.

For several months, Melinda and I had been working through The Mindful Self-Compassion Workbook by Kristin Neff. A week ago, Melinda felt like she had an "aha moment" when she read the chapter on harsh criticism. She realized that one of the reasons she stopped taking risks and stopped growing was her fear of failure. If she tried something new and it didn't work or meet her perfectionistic standards, she knew her inner critic would scold her unmercifully. Her self-critic kept her in her place. It kept her in her dilemma.

At this point, I knew we needed to try a new strategy. She needed something positive to overcome and rebalance the overwhelming distress in her life. She needed an inner source of light that could motivate and point the way to a fresh, inspiring path. I decided it was a good time to reintroduce Melinda to her natural giftedness. Starting with the earliest memories she could recall then progressing to the present, I asked her to tell me stories of when she had accomplished things she felt were noteworthy. These stories were about tasks that she felt she was both good at and internally motivated to do. I explained to her that in activities like these we become so lost in the task at hand that we often lose sense of both time and our surroundings.

At first, she wasn't sure what I meant. She told me a story about a dance contest she won and the joy she felt when her parents praised her for winning. She felt loved and appreciated. She felt special, but it wasn't about dancing. She didn't even like dancing that much. She liked the external praise of her parents. I explained I was looking for stories of activities she enjoyed doing whether anybody witnessed them or not. We were looking for her giftedness, which is a combination of her abilities and motivations.

Her lips inched into a smile and she began to tell the story about an art contest she had won in the first grade. She remembered that as a little girl she often lost herself in drawing and painting. She would spend hours in her room making art, often forgetting to even eat.

It didn't matter what she was painting, the ability to transfer to canvas what she saw in her mind was fascinating. It was a compulsion. She loved experimenting with colors, textures and different media. Her work often took on an abstract appearance that stirred thrilling emotions inside her. Even as a little girl, she knew she was different from her siblings in this way. She knew she was good at art long before anybody told her.

As she began to recount stories of her high school experiences, her face became even more animated. She was known as the person to go to if any type of promotional artwork needed to be created: pep rally posters, student government campaign posters, fundraising banners. She even told me about how teachers and school administrators asked her to create teaching and marketing materials for the school.

In college she studied graphic design and marketing, and found the coursework fascinating. Upon graduation, she opened her own marketing company in the small town where she grew up. For several years, she grew and ran her thriving business. She energetically told me stories of the marketing campaigns she ran and the companies she represented. She became especially spirited when she told me about a logo she created for a local grocery store. She recalled that every time her mother visited the grocery store, she would pridefully point out to the manager, bag boy or cashier that her daughter had designed their logo. It was obvious that she was good at what she did and enjoyed it immensely.

In her early thirties, she met the man she wanted to marry and felt it was time to take a different path. She decided to focus on raising her family. She closed her creative design company. She continued to draw and paint for a few years, but then life just got busy and her art studio gathered dust. "And now," she said, "I am where I am." It felt like all the energy had been sucked out of the room. Her countenance, which had been gregarious and glowing only moments before, now fell flat and despondent.

The contrast in her mood and expression was amazing, but even more amazing was the fact that she didn't recognize it. I confronted her and asked if she realized what had just happened. She was oblivious.

As I mentioned earlier, for time and simplicity I have only provided a small portion of Melinda's entire interview and will skip directly to identifying the patterns of her stories. You may find it helpful, however, to make a separate copy of the Story Note form for each of Melinda's stories and identify the five story elements for each of them first. This is what I recommend you do for your own stories. Once you have done that, proceed to identifying the patterns. You can see an example of what Melinda's completed Story Pattern form looks like in Figure 5.9.

MELINDA'S STORY PATTERNS

Abilities: *action words, verbs*	drawing, painting, create, studied, opened, grew, and ran
Subject Matter: *objects of people that you worked on, with, or through*	colors, textures, canvas, paint, pencils, "different mediums," visions in my head, abstractions, promotional work, pep rally posters, fundraising banners, teaching materials, marketing materials, graphic design, marketing, thriving marketing business, grocery store logo
Circumstances: *setting, environment, conditions, triggers, motivations*	art contest; invited by teachers and fellow students to create; school work; defined projects, completed tasks
Role: *how you interacted or related to others*	solitary
Satisfaction: *what you found satisfying about the activity*	emotionally thrilling to create on paper what I saw in my head, mother's praise, seeing her work in public, helping people succeed

(FIGURE 5.9)

MELINDA'S GIFTEDNESS SUMMARY STATEMENT

Melinda is an artistic creative who loves translating her visions into tangible objects in order to help promote and improve other people's lives, work and missions.

Melinda was stuck in a gray and sterile world doing somebody else's work. I suggested that she begin reclaiming her life by reintroducing a bit of creative color. Reopening her home studio and dedicating a little time to painting would be a good start. Just the thought of the possibility brought a smile back to her face.

She may never make her living using her creative gifts again, but the point wasn't about making a living. She needed to rediscover how to make a life. Painting, drawing and creating weren't an option for her. They were a need; a compulsion that demanded her attention. She thought she could ignore them, but in doing so she ignored the very thing that fueled her meaning, growth and fulfillment. She was created for that purpose.

As Melinda began to incorporate her natural gifts back into her life, she infused the uncomfortable tasks of daily living with energizing purpose. She felt more empowered and, as predicted, both her confidence and motivation improved. As she reclaimed her gifts, she reclaimed the other areas of her life: her marriage, her career, her emotional health, and her physical health.

Summary

1. People who live life well place more emphasis on strengthening their inherit assets that trying to fortify their weaknesses.

2. Your assets are the combination of your unique strengths and the things that you are naturally interested in doing.

3. Growth and progressively living a better life come as a function of two elements:

a. Developing a strong set of skills or tools to handle adversity.

b. Matching your skill set with your challenges, implying that you must allow yourself to face adversity.

4. Recognizing and acknowledging your inherent strengths encourages and motivates you to assume new challenges. New successes then breed more success.

5. Because you have never lived without your assets, it can be difficult for you to recognize them.

6. Methods for identifying your inherent assets:

   a. Strengths identification sheet

   b. Aptitude or Personality Testing

      i. Big Five Personality Traits

      ii. Myers-Briggs Type Indicator

      iii. DiSC

      iv. StrengthsFinder

      v. Enneagram

7. Because humans primarily use story to help us understand our environment and circumstances, story is an ideal method to help you understand your own assets.

8. Your giftedness revealed through story:

   a. List your stories

   b. Write or tell your stories

   c. Analyze your stories

   d. Look for patterns

   e. Consolidate your stories into a single summary statement

So far you have learned how the stories of your past behaviors shed light on your innate **Assets**, how **Awareness** of your internal characters (your emotions) can help you drive your present and future stories in more positive directions, and how **Attenuating** the volume of your internal negative thoughts can help you understand your unmet needs and provide for them in healthier ways. In the next chapter, I will discuss ways you can intentionally design and choose environments so they become **Allies** in your journey to living well.

CHAPTER 6

Allies — Cultivate Positive Enriching Relationships & Environments

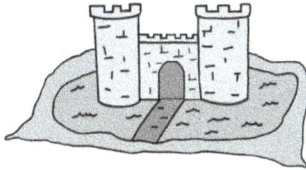

ARRIVAL GATE 1A: Adversity

DEPARTURE GATE 6A: Awareness, Attenuation, Assets, Allies, Aim, Action

Boarding Pass	Empowered Self-Care	Boarding Pass
Username: _____	**First Class**	← ☑ Departures
Destination: Beautiful Life	Current Location: Reality	✈ **6A**
Arrival: **Gate 1A** (Adversity)		Gate
Departure: **Gate 6A** (Awareness, Attenuation, Assets, Allies, Aim, Action)		

Most people think: that they act autonomously,
with minimal influence from external factors.

The truth is: your environment, especially the people you surround yourself with, influences your behavior much more than you realize. We all need fortifications of enriched nurturing relationships to help protect and encourage us during life's adversities as well as to share in our moments of happiness and accomplishments.

"Much was possible to a man in solitude. [...] But some things were possible only to a man in companionship, and of these the most important was balance. No mind was so good that it did not need another mind to counter and equal it, and to save it from conceit and blindness and bigotry and folly."[60]

"Plant yourself in a tall forest if you hope to have ideas of stature."[61]

I n 1916 Ronald, a recent college graduate with a degree in English, found himself slogging through the mud- and disease-infested trenches of France during WWI as a second lieutenant in the British Expeditionary Force. Rotting food, marauding rats, decaying bodies, festering wounds, blood sucking lice, and burning gunpowder replaced his picturesque Oxford University campus. Ronald was a heady dreamer, the antithesis of the strong warrior type, who now found himself conscripted in this godforsaken place. Four weeks into the Battle of the Somme, Ronald was embroiled in one of history's bloodiest fights. Over three million men fought in the battle and approximately one million were wounded or killed. Fighting for every inch, on one side lay the Allied forces of France and England and on the other the troops of Germany. In between lay a vast wasteland of mud, barbed wire, corpses, and bomb craters. The forest had been decimated, its few remaining trees left standing as haggard, spiked posts stripped of their great green cloaks. Nothing lived in No Man's Land.Wave upon wave of young Allied soldiers were mowed down by the strafing of German

60 Charles Williams, *Charles Williams: Collected Works* (Kindle Editions, 2015).

61 Karen Burke LeFevre, *Invention as a Social Act* (Carbondale: Southern Illinois University Press, 1987).

machine guns. It seemed pointless. The zigzagged trenches designed to protect and shield paradoxically morphed into elongated mass graves, entombing a generation of young men. As his external world reeled in chaos, Ronald retreated into the recesses of his imagination, into a world that he'd begun creating as a small child. Some had accused him of using his imaginative worlds as an escape, but they misunderstood. Writing was his attempt, both in the moment and years later, to make sense of the horrific carnage and to give it meaning.

Ronald was born in South Africa to his mother Mabel and father Arthur who were both British. His father sailed to South Africa to discover riches, and in the process found a lucrative job as an assistant bank manager for the Bank of Africa in the Free State of South Africa. His mother hated the isolation, wild animals and heat of Africa. She longed for the comforts of England. Fearing for Ronald's health after he was bitten by a large spider, Mabel returned to England with her children, leaving Arthur in Africa. A few months later, Arthur contracted rheumatic fever and died. Ronald was only four.

Mabel, looking for a more tranquil place to recover and raise her small boys, settled in a rural community near Birmingham, England. The rolling hills, meadows, ponds, streams, and forests of this quiet, agrarian community made an ideal setting for young, curious boys to explore and play. This idyllic home felt comfortable and safe. It became the home of his imaginative worlds to which he could return whenever his external world turned threatening. Mabel encouraged her sons to independently explore and roam in the outdoors. She also urged them to explore the potentials of their minds, sharing with them her love for learning and the arts. In addition to various African dialects and languages they had been exposed to in Bloemfontein, Mabel taught the boys German, French and Latin. Learning language syntax was just an academic stepping stone, however. The real prize lay in the power of words to create story, move emotion and capture dreams. She introduced them to classic works like Alice's Adventures in Wonderland, The Princess and the Goblin, and The Princess and Curdie. Ronald was a natural with words with a vivid imagination, and he began creating his own languages and stories at an early age.

Not knowing what other natural gifts her children may have, Mabel nurtured not only language, but the arts of calligraphy, drawing and painting. Equipped now with a wide arsenal of tools, Ronald reached deep into his imagination to bring his creations to life with a multisensory narration of words and non-phonetic visual languages. For the remainder of his life, Ronald punctuated his stories with his unique and cryptic watercolor paintings.

In 1900, Mabel and her sister converted to Catholicism for reasons unknown. This was no insignificant matter, since doing this in England at the time was tantamount to heresy. She was ostracized by the remainder of her family. Her husband's meager estate quickly dwindled and the family moved from the angelic shire to one dreary residence after another. The church introduced turmoil to their lives, but it also provided tangible relief. Father Francis Xavier Morgan descended on the family like a benevolent godfather. He offered them financial assistance and became a role model for Mabel's boys. Ronald recalls that it was Father Francis who taught him the meaning of charity and forgiveness.

When Ronald was twelve years old, his mother died from diabetes. She was only thirty-four. Father Francis and Ronald's aunt were the only two people at her bedside. Ronald wrote to his own son, Christopher, in 1941 as he remembered his mother, "Gifted lady of great beauty and wit, greatly stricken by God with grief and suffering, who died in youth of a disease hastened by persecution of her faith."[62] In his mind, she was a martyr for her faith and the cruelty of her family only strengthened his resolve to follow in her brave steps.

---

62 Philip Zaleski and Carol Zaleski, *The Fellowship: The Literary Lives of the Inklings* (Farrar, Straus and Giroux, 2015).

Fate cast upon Ronald at such an early age the strident polarity of extremes: love and loneliness, happiness and despair, comfort and need. Deeply rooted in his Catholic faith, Ronald's morality drew stark contrasts between right and wrong, good and evil. It must have seemed that the idyllic countryside and its simple yet honest life, a devoted mother and the father figure of Father Francis came at a high cost.

Electrical currents flow from positive to negative. Heat flows from hot to cold, and storms from high pressure to low pressures. Polarized emotions create similar currents and demand an outlet. For some it's exercise. For others it is eating. Yet others bury themselves in work or turn to drugs and alcohol. Ronald focused his energy ever deeper into creating his internal mystical worlds.

The British army noted Ronald's skill for languages and recruited him to encode military messages. Because field phone lines could easily be tapped, they most often used carrier pigeons, flares or soldiers to carry messages. Even in this less dangerous capacity, the life expectancy of new recruits on the frontline was less than two weeks. Exploding bombs and ricocheting bullets only reinforced his childhood notion that the world was divided into stark contrasting forces of good and evil.

Within him, his stories personified the dichotomy of his external worlds. One world was filled with peaceful, curious and brave inhabitants reminiscent of his idyllic childhood home. The other world was a dark dangerous place filled with death, fear, disease, and loneliness—a place where the sun was afraid to shine and the abusers of mankind ruled with no mercy.

England was embroiled in the fight for its life. Ronald felt that the country needed its own epic mythology, a mythology that—while not overtly Christian—held true to its core tenants. Ordinary people needed a mythology that emboldened and empowered them to do noble deeds. Ronald didn't believe, as with the ancient Greek myths, that courageous acts could only be accomplished by a select chosen few. He saw bravery every day on the battlefront, in the acts of young men and lowly privates who braved the onslaught of evil despite facing the ultimate sacrifice. He saw courage in a poor widow who refused to bow to the pressures of society and forsake her beliefs. He saw courage in a young mother who, despite monetary poverty, refused to allow her children to succumb to poverty of the mind. Ronald believed in an honest style of bravery and courage for which we all can strive and hope. Ronald believed that the best example of bravery is knowing not only when to fight but when to forgive.

One of his characters speaks of his heart better than I can:

"(The antagonist of the story) believes that it is only a great power that can hold evil in check, but that is not what I have found. I found it is the small things, everyday deeds of ordinary folk, that keeps the darkness at bay, simple acts of kindness and love."

"True courage is about knowing not when to take a life but when to spare one."[63]

In October of 1916, Ronald contracted trench fever, a severe, lice-borne disease, and was shipped back to England to recover. His time in the war ended, but the indelible mark it left on his consciousness and his life's work was permanent.

Ten years later, Ronald began teaching English language and literature at Pembroke College at Oxford University. It was during this tenure that he met Clive Staples at a faculty meeting. Clive was a fellow at nearby Magdalen College, and was teaching the same subjects as Ronald. Even though both loved the art of language, they clashed.

---

63 Peter Jackson, *The Hobbit: An Unexpected Journey* [Film] (Metro-Goldwyn-Mayer (MGM), New Line Cinema, WingNut Films, 2012).

In his diary, Clive described Ronald as, "A smooth, pale, fluent little chap [...] No harm in him: only needs a smack or so."[64]

Ronald was Catholic and Clive an atheist. Ronald argued that Oxford's English curriculum should emphasize the origin of language, otherwise known as philology. Clive, on the other hand, fought for the side of classic literature. Words to Clive were mere tools entrusted to carry the story.

In an attempt to win support for his cause, Ronald founded a club called the Kolbitar to foster love for ancient literature and languages. ("Kolbiter" is a medieval Norwegian word for "Coal biters," meaning a group of men who would sit around a fire so closely it looked like they were biting the coals.) Clive joined and was immediately hooked.

With time, the two became inseparable and together changed the face of English Literature. As you may have already guessed, Ronald's full name was John Ronald Reuel Tolkien, better known as J.R.R. Tolkien, author of *The Hobbit* and *The Lord of the Rings* trilogy. You know Clive Staples as C.S. Lewis, author of *The Chronicles of Narnia*, *The Screwtape Letters* and *Mere Christianity*.

In December of 1929, three years after their initial meeting, Tolkien shared with Clive a draft of a poem he had written, *The Lay of Leithian*. This marked the first time he had shown anyone his stories other than his high school English teacher. It was a love story between a mortal man, Beren, who fled the Battle of Sudden Flame and escaped into the world of elves. Here he fell in love with a beautiful elf named Lúthien Tinuviel. According to scholars, it is one of Tolkien's most personal stories.

Intimate relationships can only begin when one party allows themselves to become vulnerable to the other. The image is of a subject bowing before a king. By doing so, they expose the back of their

---

64   C. S. Lewis, *All My Road Before Me: The Diary of C. S. Lewis, 1922-1927* (Harper One. Reprint Edition, February 14, 2017).

neck, in effect saying, "I make myself vulnerable to your desires. If you deem my life unworthy, then my neck is bare to your sword." Tolkien took this brave step and allowed himself to become bare to Lewis's critique.

Lewis was enthralled with the poem, writing to Tolkien, "I can quite honestly say that it is ages since I have had an evening of such delight: and the personal interest of reading a friend's work had very little to do with it. I should have enjoyed it just as well as if I'd picked it up in a bookstop, by an unknown author." He warned however, "Detailed criticisms will follow."[65]

The way Lewis shrouded his critique in his inventive story likely removed some of the sting and made the critique less personal. Lewis created a panel of fictitious scholars named Pumpernickel, Peabody, Schick, Bentley, and Schuffer, who each wrote critical reviews of the piece. This was extensive, and Lewis even took the audacious move of rewriting entire passages.

Tolkien loved it. Impressed with Lewis's ingenious approach, Tolkien incorporated many of his suggestions. "Almost all the verses which Lewis found wanting," Tolkien's son Christopher wrote, "for one reason or another are marked for revision [...] if not actually rewritten, and in many cases his proposed emendations, or modifications of them, are incorporated in the text."[66] In the late 1950s, Tolkien was still rewriting the poem and considering Lewis's original critique.

For any new relationship to take root, however, vulnerability must be reciprocal. Lewis followed Tolkien's lead by sharing some of his original poems, and the nidus for the Inklings was born.

---

65 Philip Zaleski and Carol Zaleski, *The Fellowship: The Literary Lives of the Inklings* (Farrar, Straus, and Girou, 2015).

66 Diana Pavalac Glyer, Bandersnatch: *C. S. Lewis, J. R. R. Tolkien, and the Creative Collaboration of the Inklings* (Black Squirrel Books, 2016).

To say the effect this relationship had on the two men and the world around them was monumental is an understatement. It reached far beyond the realms of their writings. The nature of the English curriculum at Oxford University was influenced as Lewis adopted Tolkien's love for the root of language. The friendship led to the conversion of Lewis from atheism to theism and eventually Lewis accepted Christianity as a "true myth."[67]

The Inklings started small with a simple agenda. Meet every Thursday night, typically at Lewis's apartment, drink hot tea and smoke pipes. C.S. Lewis would then exclaim, "Well has anybody got anything to read us?" Some brave soul would read their recent work and they would "settle down to sit in judgement upon it."[68] The Inklings were supportive, but scathing in their assessments.

In addition to the formal meetings at Lewis's house, the Inklings often met more casually at a local pub, The Eagle and Child, which they called "The Bird and Baby."

But for the efforts of Lewis and the other Inklings, Tolkien would have never completed *The Lord of the Rings*. Before meeting Lewis, Tolkien was known for his "children's book," *The Hobbit*, but he was floundering for new ideas for its sequel. Tolkien lost himself in endless passages of Hobbit language while the movement of the storyline fell stagnant. As a part of his usual weekly meeting with the Inklings, Tolkien read chapters from this new sequel. Lewis did not like the direction Tolkien was taking. He suggested that he should simplify the language and create more movement in the story. Lewis advised that everything of interest that happens to the Hobbits should occur outside of the Shire.

---

67 Diana Pavalac Glyer, Bandersnatch: *C. S. Lewis, J. R. R. Tolkien, and the Creative Collaboration of the Inklings* (Black Squirrel Books, 2016).

68 Philip Zaleski and Carol Zalesk, *The Fellowship: The Literary Lives of the Inklings* (Farrar, Straus, and Giroux, 2015).

With a new vision and spark, the sequel to *The Hobbit* became England's greatest mythologic quest, *The Lord of the Rings*.

As you look at Tolkien's life through the lens of history, it seems obvious how his early childhood home, the love of his mother, his mother's faith, the trenches of WWI, and the Inklings heavily shaped his work. You and I are not immune to these types of influences either. Eventually, people will look at your life and it will be just as obvious how experiences, trials, environments, and people influenced your work. You can either harness these forces to help you achieve something great, or you can passively drift wherever they lead.

As with Tolkien, you may not always be able to control your circumstances. Your early childhood is determined by your parents' lives. Your environment may continue to be controlled by others even as you age. Tolkien was conscripted into a war he did not choose. You can learn from Tolkien, however. Unlike many others, once he broke free from the tyranny of war, he chose to surround himself with the great thinkers of Oxford University, a nurturing environment for his talents. When the opportunity arose, he sought Allies. He didn't passively succumb to fate; he organized his own alliances—initially the Kolbiters, then the Inklings.

Allies are all of the collaborative positive forces you can call upon to help mold your automatic biases, beliefs and behaviors. They include the environments, systems, circumstances, and people with which you surround yourself. In the western world, and especially in the US, we like to think of ourselves as lone agents who act independently, but the truth is that we all are influenced in ways we don't completely understand, in ways that remain invisible to our conscious self.

Types of Allies

The heroes of both Tolkien and Lewis, unlike the lone heroes of modern stories, were not solitary actors. Their protagonists built complex and diverse alliances. Like them, your greatest allies are the people with whom you associate. They can be classified into six broad categories. Your situation will determine which type of Ally best serves you. Most often, the best answer is a combination. As your situation changes, so will the type of assistance you need.

1. Supporters are individual acquaintances, friends or family who provide encouragement and assistance. You should recruit these individuals as early as possible. Interested only in your wellbeing, their support comes free. They are an excellent source of encouragement. Their expertise in your desired area of growth, however, may be limited. Because they may fear harming the relationship, they may not hold you as accountable as you need, and they may refrain from honest criticisms which could be helpful to your growth.

2. Masterminds are small groups of people who meet regularly to encourage, assist and hold each other accountable. The people of your mastermind need not have any expertise, training or experience in your area of interest. Masterminds can be guided by a central leader or not. I like to think of masterminds as a roundtable of allies. It is a group of equals. Nobody has any more authority or skill than anybody else. Each person contributes equally to propagate the journey of its individual members. The Inklings are an example of this type of roundtable. They refined and purified each other's work. I have found that masterminds are one of the best ways to foster personal creativity, promote accountability and nurture growth. The price of membership into a mastermind group can range from free to expensive. We will discuss how to organize and run your own roundtable alliance later in the chapter.

3. Mentors have no formal training or significant experience in a field of interest, but walk a few steps ahead of you on a similar path. They willingly share what they have experienced and learned. Typically, mentors share one-on-one. Most often, mentors freely share their experiential wisdom when they find an apprentice who is willing to learn and take action. Let me repeat: Mentors share only to the extent that you are willing to learn and enact. Once you implement their suggestions, report back with your results. Mentors are energized by your action. The relationship is not guaranteed, however, and is dependent on their willingness to freely share.

4. **Coaches** have formal training or moderate experience in a given field, but are not considered experts. They primarily help people maximize their innate potential. Coaches can work with both individuals and groups. They charge a fee for their time. Because your relationship is contractually determined, you are guaranteed access to them. Before you hire a coach, make sure you clearly understand the extent of the support and services they provide. Search for a coach that augments your personality style. Clearly communicate with them how you like to communicate and be held accountable, i.e. some people respond to words of encouragement, others prefer a more aggressive, in-your-face approach.

5. **Professors** are considered experts in their field, either through extensive formal training or through their work in a specified field. They may be found in a university or other higher education setting. They simply disseminate knowledge; they do not help people implement information. Professors teach directly through lectures and writings, as well as indirectly through their life story. Because you can read a professor's cognitive work after they die, they continue to teach posthumously. Consuming information from professors can greatly reduce your learning time. Reading is an excellent way to learn from the great professors of history as well as contemporary experts. Because the venues through which professors teach are so diverse, the cost of their services can be small—as in the price of a book—to more substantial—as in the cost of a seminar or a formal course.

6. **Professor Coaches** are a rare breed. They are the few experts who not only disseminate knowledge, but also support and encourage people while they implement the information. Professor coaches,

because of the demand for their time and expertise, charge a premium. If you have adequate time and money, this is the most effective way to maximize your growth curve.

Most people seek help too late in their journey. They wait until they are completely overwhelmed. You should intentionally seek support from the beginning. Overwhelm creeps up quickly and without warning. Negative messages arise automatically. They need no encouragement and, as you learned earlier, they carry more weight than your positive encouraging voices.

Start simple. Share your task with a friend. Reach out to a mentor and offer to buy them lunch in exchange for their advice. Pick up a biography of one of history's great leaders. Commit to reading just a few pages a day. Note what they did differently from ordinary people. Apply those lessons to your own life.

Start Small and Seek Help

Admiral William H. McRaven delivered a commencement speech at the University of Texas in May of 2014. At the time I wrote this book, over 25 million people have viewed it on YouTube. His book, *Make Your Bed,* expounds on the principles of his speech and the lessons he learned during Navy Seal training. The subtitle captures his central message, "Little Things That Change Your Life ... And Maybe the World."

When people look at the gargantuan accomplishments of their heroes, they believe the keys to success must be proportional to the size of their great feats. We naturally compare ourselves to our heroes. We attempt to emulate them. When we focus on the scale of their accomplishments, however, we become overwhelmed. The truth is, their success was built on small things that they consistently linked together. Focus not on your heroes' end results, but on the small steps that led to their success. Focus on your own small steps, and this similar approach can result in successful living or progressively growing along your unique life path.

McRaven's first two lessons are most applicable for our discussion:

1. Make your bed every morning. Start your day with a task accomplished. Success creates an attitude of success. Accomplishment breeds a mindset of accomplishment. Stop waiting for somebody else to fix your problems. Take intentional steps to heal yourself. Admiral McRaven shares, "Making my bed correctly was not going to be an opportunity for praise. It was expected of me. It was my first task of the day, and doing it right was important. It demonstrated my discipline. It showed my attention to detail, and at the end of the day it would be a reminder that I had done something well, something to be proud of, no matter how small the task."[69]

Truthfully, I've never been one to make my bed. I hate to sleep in a neat bed, so it seems pointless. Reading and writing are my tasks to accomplish. I decided that I wanted to learn from the great minds of history. Every morning, I wake up around 4:00 a.m. (5:00 a.m. on weekends) to read, write, pray, and meditate for three or four hours. These hours set the tone for the rest of my day. I read about ancient philosophers like Aristotle, Plato and Socrates. I read the biographies and autobiographies of great leaders and thinkers such as Benjamin Franklin, Michelangelo, Albert Einstein, and Winston Churchill. I read science journal articles and textbooks. I read ancient wisdom literature and Christian scripture. My philosophy of science and religion is similar to the late Sir William Henry Bragg, "From religion comes a man's purpose; from science, his power to achieve it. Sometimes people ask if religion and science are not opposed to one another. They are: in the sense that the thumb and fingers of my hands are opposed to one another. It is an opposition by means of which anything can

---

69 William H. McRaven, *Make Your Bed: Little Things That Can Change Your Life ... And Maybe The World*, (Grand Central Publishing, 2017).

be grasped."[70] I have made it my life's endeavor to study at the feet of history's great professors.

Are you beginning your day with a task accomplished? What can you do to start your day with a positive achievement? Begin with a small step. I managed this by waking up five minutes early and it grew from there. Five minutes led to ten minutes, then thirty minutes, then an hour, then finally three hours. In essence, it only took five minutes to change the trajectory of my life. What minimal step can you take that could change your life? From what great professors, coaches or mentors can you learn?

2. Find somebody to help you paddle. Nobody lives successfully without the help of other people. Navy Seals in training, otherwise known as "tadpoles," are assigned to a ten-foot rubber raft along with six other tadpoles. They are required to take the raft everywhere. They take it to the chow hall. They run with it up and down the sand dunes of Coronado beach. They paddle it up and down the coastline. Eventually, somebody gets hurt or sick, yet training continues. As the sick or injured stumble and weaken, the other six shoulder their burden until they recover. McRaven comments, "The small rubber boat made us realize that no man could make it through combat alone and, by extension, you needed people in your life to help you through the difficult times [...] None of us are immune to life's tragic moments."[71] Who are your supporters? Do you have a group of Inklings to chide you on? When you get injured and become discouraged, do you have somebody who will share your burden? The counterpoint is applicable as well: who are you supporting?

---

70 Abdus Salam, *The Art of the Physicist*, New Scientist, Vol. 35 (20 Jul 1967), 163.

71 William H. McRaven, *Make Your Bed: Little Things That Can Change Your Life ... And Maybe The World* (Grand Central Publishing, 2017).

A New Creative Ally

In 2014, I started writing a blog. Blogging was popular, but not many physicians were doing it. Other than scientific papers, I hadn't written anything since college, and I didn't know anything about creating a blog, email lists, a website or landing pages. While I may not have known much about writing, I did know that action begets action, so I just started writing. Slowly, and I must admit a little painfully, I learned. My first blog post was a disaster. I misused the word "elusion" when I meant to use "illusion." No big deal, you say, but it was the central premise of my article. I almost didn't write another post, but I pressed on.

A business coach I was working with, Adam Brantley, recommended that I talk to Jeff Goins, an author from Nashville, who was starting a mastermind group for aspiring writers, called Tribe Writers Pro. After visiting Jeff, he offered me the last of twelve spots. I eagerly accepted.

I had read about mastermind groups, but had never been part of one.

The first time I encountered the term mastermind was when I read *Think and Grow Rich* by Napoleon Hill. Hill coined the term and defined it as, "Coordination of knowledge and effort, in a spirit of harmony, between two or more people, for the attainment of a definite purpose."[72] He claimed that Andrew Carnegie, the Steel Baron, was his inspiration for the term. Carnegie surrounded himself with a "staff" of people for the express purpose of generating ideas, or what Hill called "thought-energy." Hill compared it to connecting batteries together in such a way that their collective power is greater than the power of any single battery. In his book he explains, "When a group

---

72 Napoleon Hill, *Think and Grow Rich* (Simon and Brown, This edition 2010, First Copyright 1937).

of individual brains are coordinated and function in harmony, the increased energy created through that alliance becomes available to every individual brain in the group."[73] I wanted to be part of something like that.

Straight out of college, Jeff joined "Adventures in Missions," a not-for-profit, nondenominational mission organization that promoted short-term missions. He was hired to market the company, but felt he was meant to do something else. On his boss's suggestion, Jeff joined a support group for burned-out youth ministers. A member of the group asked Jeff, "What is your dream?" Jeff stammered, "I mean—I suppose, I hope to maybe be a writer." His friend responded, "You don't have to want to be a writer. You are a writer. You just need to write." The next day, Jeff started his blog. A year later, he quit his job and wrote his first book, *Wrecked*, in 2012. He describes it as a trans-formative experience, "Everybody but me knew that I was a writer. I was very scared to make that transition."[74] He published his second book, *You Are a Writer (So Start acting Like One)* in 2014. One simple question from a friend changed the entire direction of his life.

After Jeff quit his job, a photographer friend asked him to join a new mastermind group he was starting. Jeff's friend and two other young businessmen had recently read *Think and Grow Rich* and had decided to start their own mastermind. Twelve guys ultimately joined and met weekly on Wednesday mornings from 7:00 a.m. until 8:30 a.m., ate breakfast, read a book and talked about it, shared their stories and challenges in business, and helped each other. Does this sound familiar? (Hint—Inklings.) Jeff was a part of that mastermind group for six years.

---

73   Napoleon Hill, *Think and Grow Rich* (Simon and Brown, This edition 2010, First Copyright 1937).

74   Jeff Goins, interview conducted by David W. Ball, MD. 2018.

When I contacted Jeff, he had been running an online writing course, Tribe Writers, for a couple of years and was about to release *The Art of Work,* which went on to become a *New York Times* bestseller. His course was successful, but he wanted to create a more hands-on and impactful process for struggling writers. Given the transformative impact his personal mastermind groups had on his own life, Jeff decided to start his own mastermind for writers. The small group format I joined was his first attempt to do that.

When I flew to Nashville for our first meeting, I was a bit nervous. Actually, I was way out of my comfort zone. Science, medicine and academia had been my world for the last couple of decades. What was I doing? I must have lost my mind! Who was I fooling? I wasn't a writer. I was about to walk into a room of right-brained creatives and my left brain was running scared.

The Frothy Monkey, a low-key, hip coffee house in Franklin, Tennessee, was to be our home for the next several days. It was fitting for the creative vibe Jeff was trying to achieve. It sits in the heart of old downtown Franklin, close to the square. A two-story brick building with a large, traditional, southern front porch, it is adorned with a central inviting set of stairs which leads directly to the front door. It's one of Jeff's favorite places to hang out. As I walked in, the aroma of coffee and the sound of bustling people had a familiar, comfortable feel.

I must have looked lost because a friendly barista greeted me and asked if she could help. I asked where Tribe Writers Pro was meeting, and she pointed me up a switchback staircase to the right. I slowly walked up the stairs and found the room where Jeff was standing with a couple of other people.

In the center, a circle of wooden, industrial-style tables had been set up, reminiscent of King Arthur's legendary round table. A place setting with a glass and a stack of materials was in front of each chair. To the right was a table stacked with snacks and cold drinks. As everybody trickled in, we claimed a spot at the table. Jeff introduced himself and I don't think I heard anything he said in the introduction; all I could hear was my inner voice. "What are you doing here? You're not a writer," it repeated, first softly then increasingly louder, to the point it was screaming at me. Then, as if somebody knocked me back to reality, I heard Jeff say, "You are a writer, so start acting like one." That moment was another inflection point in my life.

What a wonderful set of people I met that day. What a rejuvenating atmosphere it was. I felt myself start to relax and revitalize. Most primary care physicians I knew at the time were frustrated with the state of medicine. Many were on the verge of burnout. Any time a group of us gathered, it turned into a gripe session. We complained about malpractice. We complained about long work hours. We complained about unrealistic expectations. We complained about electronic medical records. We complained about insurance companies. It was death by a thousand cuts.

Sitting in a coffee house in Nashville, I felt inspired for the first time in ages. I felt uplifted. Everybody was so positive and excited about the future. I wasn't used to this. People were enthusiastic about what they were doing. They were excited about the possibility of accomplishing something great. Optimism and hope percolated through the room. I didn't recognize it at first, but what had been masquerading as fear was excitement and hope that a new chapter was unfolding, anticipation that the price of vulnerability would be worth the sacrifice. Like standing in a warm shower on a cold winter morning, I felt the warmth of acceptance flow across my body and melt my stoicism. I like this, I thought. I'm not sure I want to go back.

This group met formally as part of Jeff's Tribe Writer Pro program for one year, then we met independently for another year and a half. This book exists in part because of their encouragement and example.

Mastermind Principles

My experience in Nashville left me feeling that I had the responsibility to give back to others what had been given to me. While I can't invite everybody to my hometown for an intimate get-together, I can share a few recommendations and an outline that will help you build or find a successful mastermind of your own.

Ideally you would start or find a group that meets in person. To start your own group, ask a person or two you already know and think may be interested, somebody you think will bring energy and an interesting, discerning perspective. You're looking for people with an abundance mindset, who enjoy giving and sharing freely with others. If you are older and hopefully a little wiser than the younger version of yourself, this could be an opportunity to share your successes and failures with a less experienced person. Stay on the lookout for those talents in the rough. Including them in your mastermind group could be a life-changing experience. On the other hand, if you are young, inexperienced or don't feel like you are an expert at anything, don't worry. The beauty of the mastermind is that the group brings collective wisdom to the conversation. In addition, what you don't know collectively, you can learn through inviting thought leaders into the conversation.

If you don't know enough people in your circle, extend the invitation to the friends and acquaintances of the people you have already invited. If you do, make sure to clearly communicate your desired inclusion criteria. You may also want to interview the prospect before incorporating them into the group.

Don't worry about trying to create a large group. You are looking to develop deep, intimate relationships, so by nature the group will need to stay small. In the beginning you may want to keep the group to three or four people.

I would also encourage you to invite people outside your area of expertise. Diversity is important. As a physician, I would not want to invite only physicians. While we all are different people, our experience is similar enough that our perspectives may be too alike. It would be helpful to broaden the group's mix by inviting businessmen, artists, bankers, teachers, coaches, writers, clergy or athletic trainers.

You can set up your mastermind group around any number of different topics, goals, common interests or products. My mastermind group in Nashville was formed around writing. My online mastermind group formed around entrepreneurship. You could form one around growing orchids, developing a community, deepening your religious experience or simply to encourage everyone to become better versions of themselves. There is no one "right" way to do it.

If you live in a small community, or if nobody in your circle is interested, you may consider searching the internet for groups or organizations that already exist around the interest you are trying to accomplish. These groups may already have a mechanism in place to join similar small groups or have chat rooms where you can offer an invitation to start an online mastermind group. The first mastermind group I joined was an online group like this. I didn't think anybody I knew would be interested in an entrepreneur-style mastermind, so I joined an online membership-style business development group. Among the various resources it offered were online mastermind groups.

Some thought leaders have established online mastermind groups as well. Think about researching their websites or querying their organizations. If they don't offer something, they may know somebody in their field who does. They may not use the word "mastermind" specifically, but could offer support groups, mentoring groups or extended small group workshops that serve a similar purpose.

Tips for Success

1. Meet in person: Non-verbal cues are just as—or sometimes more—important than the words people use. If you cannot meet in person regularly, use some type of video conferencing application. Even if you primarily meet online, consider gathering in person a few times during the year. There is nothing like face-to-face contact to solidify relationships. My writing mastermind group met in Nashville four times a year and then every other week over Zoom.

2. Charge a membership fee: Each member should pay a fee to join. It can be as small or large as you wish. I have heard of groups charging as little as $10 a month and as much as hundreds of thousands of dollars a year. My personal experience has corroborated data suggesting that when people pay for something they value it more. You only want people who are serious about participating and growing. Use the money to help offset the cost of an out-of-town weekend retreat, pay for a speaker, cover the cost of a meal together or all the above.

3. Start small and keep it small: If you can only find one other person, start there. Limit your group size to ten or fewer. Studies suggest that as the group grows in size, people share less.

4. Meet often: Weekly is ideal. At minimum, meet at least every other week. Stay in touch between meetings for quick fixes and socialization.

5. Encourage diversity: You want members of the group to express divergent opinions. Create a judgment-free, open dynamic that encourages a free flow of ideas. Seek out members from different professions and social groups. Dr. Robert Havard, one of the Inklings, emphasized, "Our differences laid the foundation of a friendship that lasted."[75] Similarity may draw people together, but it is their diversity that fosters great creativity and progress.

6. Criticize, but be respectful: Criticize the idea, not the person. Argue about the work, but don't dismiss it. One of the issues that led to the Inkling's demise has been attributed to Hugo Dyson's harsh critique of The Lords of the Rings. He viewed the work as nonsense and complained bitterly every time Tolkien talked of hobbits, elves and orcs.

7. Hold each other accountable: Harness the power of social pressure.

8. Celebrate successes: Be sensitive to a healthy balance of encouragement with your critiques.

9. Work hard and play often: We are predominately social beings. Our greatest needs are affection and connection. We need to feel included and valued. Mastermind groups, unlike typical social groups, are powerful because they combine time focused on intentional work with time dedicated to building relationships. Strong emotional bonds strengthen the work. We respect the opinions of others more if we feel they are emotionally invested. Spend time emotionally investing in each others' lives. Part of what made the Inklings so successful was that they not only met for structured meetings in C.S. Lewis's apartment every Thursday evening, but they also frequently met less formally at the Bird and Baby. Find your own Bird and Baby to foster personal connections.

10. Start and end on time: You all are busy, so be respectful of each other's time and the intent of the group.

---

75   Diana Pavalac Glyer, Bandersnatch: *C. S. Lewis, J. R. R. Tolkien, and the Creative Collaboration of the Inklings*, (Black Squirrel Books, 2016).

Mastermind Structure

Masterminds are powerful if you follow a plan. If you don't, it will dissolve into just another social group. Social groups are fine, but if you want to push yourself to grow, be intentional.

Suggested itinerary for an hour meeting:

1. **Five minutes:** Each participant should share one win from the last week that progressed one of their goals. If they had no win, they should share something else positive they discovered, achieved, are thankful for or are excited about.

2. **Forty minutes:** The main body of the meeting can be structured in a few different ways. A good place to begin is to review a book, devote time to a discussion, bring in a speaker or listen to a recorded lecture. This gives the group time to solidify relationships before starting the main work phase of the mastermind. These topic-style reviews can also serve two other functions. They provide breaks from the main work sessions and they infuse the group with opinions and ideas from outside thought leaders.

   The main problem-solving work sessions are what set mastermind groups apart from social groups. Here, you concentrate on challenges that one or two participants are encountering. In my experience, if you have more than two participants, you will not have enough time to discuss where everybody is getting stuck each meeting—therefore, rotate. Sometimes a participant may identify a complicated obstacle that they feel may require the entire forty minutes. That's fine. Do whatever the group feels is best.

   Make sure each participant in the group comments on one positive thing and one concrete constructive suggestion the person can do to move forward. One of the beauties of a mastermind group is the diversity of strengths and perspectives that each participant brings.You want to spend enough time on each others' challenges to take advantage of that diversity.

After everybody has commented, the person presenting their challenge should summarize the opinions and state what they are going to do before the next meeting.

Version A:

Forty minutes: Book discussion, speaker/lecture, topic discussion.

Version B:

a) *Twenty minutes:* Book discussion/topic discussion.

b) *Twenty minutes:* One person explains one thing they need help with right now. The goal is to develop the very next step or steps this person needs to act upon to achieve their goal. Be specific.

Version C:

Forty minutes: One person explains one thing they need help with right now. The goal is to develop the very next step or steps this person needs to act upon to achieve their goal. Be specific.

Version D:

a) *Twenty minutes:* The first person explains one thing they need help with right now. The goal is to develop the very next step or steps this person needs to act upon to achieve their goal. Be specific.

b) *Twenty minutes:* The second person explains one thing they need help with right now. The goal is to develop the very next step or steps this person needs to act upon to achieve their goal. Be specific.

3. **Five Minutes:** Each person shares a one-sentence goal they will accomplish before the next meeting.

This totals 50 minutes, which leaves about ten minutes for 'flex' time.

Other Types of Group Alliances

I have found the mastermind structure to be the best group format for fostering personal growth because each participant rotates to the center of discussion, is held accountable to their specific goals, is encouraged, and offers a diversity of perspectives and ideas.

Other types of positive alliances also exist. If you can't find a mastermind near you, don't want to start your own or the mastermind seems too structured or aggressive for you, consider these options. If you are primarily looking for people to socialize with, think about joining a group that shares a common interest, concern or goal. Some of these groups focus solely on socializing, where others focus more on community service. Groups such as AA and other mental health therapy groups focus on self-improvement, but typically offer little personal interaction. As with mastermind groups, there is no right answer. Seek the type of group that best fits your needs at the time.

Service clubs: Service clubs are non-profit organizations where members primarily meet to do charitable work. Traditional service clubs like the Rotary Club, Lions Club and Kiwanis immediately come to mind, but thousands of other newer options exist for just about any type of work. They often play a key role in community development. While charitable work is the central focus, socialization is still one of the most important benefits of these groups.

Social clubs: Social clubs are organizations that meet around a shared interest, occupation or activity. They are quite diverse and include photography clubs, country clubs, reading clubs, chess clubs, fishing clubs or hunting clubs. While their primary focus is the common interest, they often perform charitable service work as well.

Faith-based small groups: I grew up in the Christian church. Small group meetings, or what we called Sunday school, were also a form of group alliances. The central focus was spiritual growth, but as with all these organizations, supportive relationships is also one of their key benefits. When a family member died, a loved one had surgery or I became sick, this group, in addition to my other family and friends, was among the first to respond.

Twelve-step groups: One of the most recognized groups for recovering alcoholics is Alcoholics Anonymous. Several iterations of this twelve-step style program now exist for a host of issues including eating disorders, gambling, specific drug abuse, codependency, cluttering, sex and love addicts, family disorders, debt, and workaholism. AA emphasizes a peer-to-peer mentor relationship, or what they call sponsorship, ritualized in-person meetings led by fellow participants and adherence to the central tenants, twelve steps, which encourage participants to ascribe to a broader higher ideal, assume responsibility for their own change and take concrete steps toward this.

Therapy groups: Like AA, therapy groups also help foster mental health growth, but are typically led by a mental health professional.

Building and Maintaining Healthy Relationships

Humans are primarily social/relationship-based creatures. While the focus of this book is not relationships, building and maintaining healthy relationships is primarily achieved by becoming the best version of yourself. Yes, it takes two to develop healthy relationships, but you can't force your partner or other people to change. All you can do is positively change yourself, and that is the focus of this book.

Building healthier relationships has a cyclical benefit. As you nurture your relationships, you help those you care about become better versions of themselves. As they do, these healthier roles inspire who you become. We are all influenced by the people we surround ourselves with. As the old saying goes, "Birds of a feather flock together."

Most of the top ten tools below are gleaned from data on romantic relationship research. These basic relationship principles, however, apply to any type of important connection. If you want to dig a little deeper, two of the best resources I have found are *The Seven Principles for Making Marriage Work* by John Gottman Ph.D., and *Getting the Love You Want* by Harville Hendrix Ph.D. and Helen LaKelly Hunt Ph.D.

Two things that stand in the way of us building healthy relationships:

1. **Rewards without sacrifice.** Like young children, we simply want our needs met without any work.

2. **Prisoners to the fear of change.** Our old ways of thinking and relating are more familiar and comfortable. It is easy to fear the unfamiliar. Change is uncomfortable, and it is easy to resist and even become angry at the idea of acquiring new tools for relating.

Top Ten Tools for Building and Maintaining Healthy Relationships

1. Cultivate enriching Spaces.

Imagine your relationship as a common enriching space between you and your partner. You both receive emotional nourishment from this space. You can either pollute the space with toxic attitudes, emotions and behaviors, thereby creating a wasteland of filth and garbage, or you can nurture it with respectful interactions and cultivate an enriching oasis. Both partners are responsible for the common space by eliminating toxicity to the greatest extent possible. What you choose to do decides where you emotionally dine.

Cultivating a beautiful garden requires deliberate effort. It must be tended to regularly—weeded, pruned, tilled, watered, and fertilized.

Wastelands can be the result of active malice, but most often are by-products of passive neglect, default Deep Brain automatic negative responses of blame, shame, criticism, contempt, defensiveness, and stonewalling.

Unfortunately, passive toxic attitudes and behaviors are approximately five times stronger than their more positive deliberate counterparts. For every unkind thing you say or do, you must say or do at least five kind things to return the relationship back to neutrality. If you want a vibrant, healthy and happy relationship, you must be even more intentional than that. Without intentional effort, relationships quickly deteriorate into disrepair and become undesirable places that people want to exit. If you ignore the relationship or don't respect the 5:1 negativity:positivity ratio, don't expect your partner to stay in a toxic space. That's not fair, considerate, reasonable or loving.

What does a beautiful sacred space look like to you? Set aside time for you and your partner to think and write about what your visions of this look like, then share them with each other.

2. Commit to staying in the relationship, especially in the small ways.

In the United States, almost 50 percent of married couples divorce, and many more "silently divorce." Couples silently divorce when they remain married in legal terms, yet emotionally exit the relationship.

Whether you publicly divorce your partner in court or silently divorce them by exiting the relationship in the privacy of your heart, the results are comparable.

Hendrix and Hunt have identified over 300 ways that couples exit their relationships. Here are just a few:

- Disappearing into the garage or shop
- Facebooking/social media

- Surfing the internet

- Talking on the phone

- Spending too much time with the kids

- Being wed to the computer

- Volunteering for every committee at church

- Having an affair

- Spending too much time with parents

- Falling asleep on the couch at 8:00 p.m.

- Avoiding sex

- Being sports junkies

- Four scotches a night

- Working at the office too much

- Going shopping

- Refusing to talk

- Working on the house all the time

There is nothing wrong with most of these activities (with the exception of having an affair and excessive drinking.) The problem arises in the reason you engage in the activity. If the primary reason is to avoid the relationship, you are exiting.

What ways do you silently exit your relationships? How can you intentionally turn back toward your loved ones, especially when you don't feel like it?

We exit relationships by avoiding the difficult work required to keep the sacred space between us healthy, most importantly by refusing to become a better version of ourselves. Even if we are not behaving in toxic ways, neglected spaces return to toxic chaos.

Relationships are more than managing conflict. They are about spending time with each other in mutually enjoyable activities. They are about creating positive shared memories. They are about establishing something meaningful with your limited time together.

How can you create a positive shared memory with your partner today? How can you create positive shared memories with other people you care about?

3. Prevent and manage emotional flooding.

Recognize your partner's complex nature. They are a constellation of diverse inner characters, just like you. They are not monolithic, and they are neither satan nor your savior. They are simply another human being struggling to do their best with their limited resources. Remind yourself that your partner's hurtful words and behaviors originate from only a small part of who they are; they don't define the entirety of their feelings.

Remember the lessons we learned from Dr. Gottman's Love Lab in Chapter 4: Discontinue, Distance and Distract.

First, if you begin to feel emotionally overwhelmed or flooded, clearly communicate to your partner in a non-threatening way that you need to temporarily stop the discussion.

Second, distance yourself from your partner. Go to another room or outside where you can be alone.

Third, engage in some type of soothing activity such as listening to calming music, meditating/praying, walking or reading a book.

4. First seek to understand.

As I encouraged you to do with yourself in Chapter 4, adopt an open, curious mindset rather than keeping a closed-minded, judgmental perspective. Curiosity implies humility, a recognition that no one knows everything and that you can learn something from anyone.

While it is easy to intellectually admit that you are not omniscient, it can be more difficult to emotionally respond and act in a manner consistent with that knowledge, especially when one of your more cherished perspectives is challenged. We believe the world is as we perceive it to be, and when someone challenges that, we often think they are misguided or misinformed. Curiosity, in opposition, seeks to first listen and understand.

Interestingly, becoming curious is not only the best way to understand your partner, it is one of the best ways to help your partner understand themselves. People often use conversation as a sounding board to help themselves understand what they believe and what they need. Providing your partner with space to share their thoughts helps them process what they are thinking and in turn helps you better understand their perspective. Your role is to become curious—not argue, criticize, give advice, offer information, approve, agree or even reassure. Persuasion leaves people feeling unheard, misunderstood and disrespected. They become defensive.

Dr. William R. Miller Ph.D. and Stephen Rollnick Ph.D. began developing Motivational Interviewing (MI) over thirty years ago as a means to help people understand themselves and make important changes. The premise of MI is that people already know what they need to change. The problem is not knowledge; it is ambivalence. Part of a person wants to make positive change, but another part wants to maintain the status quo. Ambivalence, with its conflict between these two opposing inner parts, is uncomfortable, so people push it out of their mind. Bringing that conflict to a conscious level is painful and can be frightening. That unwanted discomfort makes us prisoners to the fear of change. This is why we resist and even become angry at the idea of acquiring new tools for relating.

Making change is particularly difficult when it involves hardwired habits, whether they are particular behaviors or ways of thinking.

Ships are designed with a large keel to help return them to an upright position in the event a wave tilts them to one side. The measure of a ship's ability to return to its neutral, level position is called the Righting Momentum. Our internal parts act in a similar manner. If someone argues that you need to change, a "Righting Reflex" automatically engages. Their arguments act like a wave that knocks your internal system out of balance. Part of you may agree with them, but another part likely disagrees. It will resist and defend the status quo. If you want to discover, and help your partner consciously discover, what is most important to them, you need to avoid the righting reflex.

Motivational Interviewing was developed as a technique to avoid this righting reflex and help people understand themselves and others. MI is a helpful tool for psychologists and counselors to understand their clients, and it can also help you understand your partner.

Miller and Rollnick use the acronym **OARS** to introduce the initial phase of Motivational Interviewing, Engaging.

> **O:** Ask pertinent, **Open**-ended questions. Refrain from leading, close-ended questions.
>
> **A: Affirm**. As your partner shares their ideas, thoughts and concerns, note their strengths, accomplishments, positive intentions, and efforts. Intentionally look for these and bring them to your partner's attention. We all have natural strengths and assets we can use to overcome adversities. Affirming your partner's strengths will help them internalize them.
>
> **R: Reflect** what your partner says back to them. There are several ways to do this. The simplest is to repeat the words they say. Another is to offer your interpretation of what they say. "Here's what I heard ... "
>
> **S:** Condense what they say into a **Summary**. Once you finish, ask if you missed anything.

Good starting questions:

- If our efforts today were 100 percent successful, what would that look like? What would be different about our relationship?
- What might prevent us from sticking to this plan, from creating that vision?

As you reflect and summarize, make sure to provide your partner with enough space and time to process what they hear. Hearing their own thoughts spoken by another individual helps them clarify and refine what they think.

It is quite unusual for people to encounter someone who actively listens. Listening to your partner in such an intentional way is a potent tool that increases the strength of your bond. We all want and need to feel heard and understood. As you actively listen in such a profound way, you confirm that you believe they are important and what they think is meaningful. This is validating.

While actively listening validates your partner, you can be even more explicit with your acceptance. View your partner's thoughts from their perspective, especially when you disagree with them. Acknowledge how someone could come to a different, but rational, conclusion from yours. Support the validity of their autonomy and perspective by responding, "That makes sense to me," or, "I see how you could come to that conclusion."

As you continue to invest in understanding your partner, they will begin to share more freely and deeply. As they do, pay attention to what they value most, as well as their dreams and goals. If your partner doesn't explicitly share these, consider inviting them to explore them with you.

5. Make and receive repair attempts.

Pay attention to your partner's attempts to repair the relationship and be willing to receive them, even when they are partial or clumsy. Equally important, make deliberate efforts of your own.

You may consider developing and agreeing upon clear, predetermined phrases or actions that communicate your desire to repair the relationship. This helps ensure that you and your partner recognize each other's efforts.

6. Focus on becoming a better version of yourself.

Make sure the person you are becoming is congruent with your most important values. It's easier to point to other people's faults than to do the difficult work of correcting your own issues. Only once you have cleaned up your own backyard should you attempt to clean up somebody else's.

What does a better version of yourself look like to you? What does a better version of yourself look like for your partner? Share some of the specific changes you are working on that will make your partner's life better.

7. Become the primary provider for your own needs.

Find healthy ways apart from your partner to meet your own needs. Assume the responsibility of becoming your own primary care provider. Your partner is not capable of meeting all your needs and may not even clearly understand what your needs are. Your partner is also struggling to meet their own needs, just like the rest of us. They likely don't have the energy or resources to take care of you full-time. As you provide for your own needs, your partner can assume the healthier realistic role of becoming a secondary resource for your needs.

8. *Ask for what you need.*

Despite your best efforts, you will sometimes need help. That is one of the benefits of close relationships. However, your partner is not all-knowing. If you don't communicate concisely and in a constructive way, your partner will never know what you need. By communicating non-confrontationally, you continue to assume your responsibility for your needs while taking positive action to solve them.

Practical tips: Speak candidly and frankly while simultaneously doing these.

a. Speak in terms of "I" not "you." Using "I" phrases continues to focus the primary responsibility on you. Using "you" phrases connotes blame and will likely make your partner feel defensive.

b. Acknowledge your role in the problem: "I share some responsibility in … " or, "I am partially to blame … "

c. Explain how you feel, don't attack. "Here's how I feel … " "This makes me feel … " When you said … it made me feel … "

d. Speak about a specific situation and describe the facts about what happened without passing judgment.

e. State your need in positive terms. "Here's what I need … " not, "I don't want you to … "

It's not reasonable to expect your partner to know what you need if you haven't done the work to discover it yourself.

Suppressing your needs because you think they are not important or too uncomfortable to address is not the loving, respectful thing to do. This is passive and easy. It eventually breeds resentment, creating emotional distance and more toxic problems for the future. Address problems in a timely manner and don't let them linger. Sometimes the most loving thing to do is to have hard conversations.

Keep your sacred space healthy by communicating your needs clearly and in a timely manner.

9. Face your unsolvable problems.

You and your partner have different life experiences and unique gifts, so your perspectives will be different in many ways. Some arguments will arise from fundamental differences that are not solvable. While these problems may not be "solvable," you can seek to understand and respect your partner's perspective. Ignoring these types of problems, however, will not make them go away—in fact this will likely exacerbate any underlying animosity.

These intransigent problems are typically emotionally polarizing and difficult to address with empathy. How you non-verbally communicate while discussing these issues can be even more important than the words you use. Intonation, facial expressions and body language that convey contempt negate positive words and communicate disrespect. To help guide the discussion in a productive manner, you may find it helpful to recruit a non-biased mediator to intervene. This could be another family member, a friend, a pastor or a counselor.

According to Dr. Gottman, perpetual disagreements most often arise from the deep-seated needs and dreams the other may not be aware of, has never acknowledged or doesn't respect. If you find yourself in this situation, first go back to tip #4 and seek to understand.

When fundamental dreams and needs are not met or respected, you will find yourself continuously battling over them either explicitly or implicitly. Superficial arguments like, for example, how to cook eggs in the morning become battles about much deeper issues.

With unsolvable problems the goal is not to win. Neither of you must give in or lose, but you must acknowledge and discuss them with respect.

10. *Become your partner's unconditional advocate.*

Intentionally cherish your partner. Remind yourself and your partner of their positive characteristics, values, strengths, and assets. Make a list of them and read them daily. Our attention is automatically drawn to people's faults. You must be more intentional about focusing on your partner's assets. As we discussed earlier, you can't become an advocate for what you don't know, therefore you must dedicate time and effort into understanding first. Become a lifelong student of your partner. Affirm your partner's strengths, achievements, good intentions, and positive efforts.

Conclusion

In *The Fellowship Of the Ring*, Frodo laments, "I wish the ring had never come to me. I wish none of this had happened."[76] His words ring eerily similar to Christ's prayer in the Garden of Gethsemane, "If it be possible, let this cup pass from me."[77] All of us will experience a time when we wish the cup could pass from us. As if knowing we too will ask for such a reprieve, Gandolf replies, "So do all who live to see such times, but that is not for them to decide. All we have to decide is what to do with the time that is given us. There are other forces at work in this world beside the will of evil."[78]

Some criticize the Inklings for wasting their time creating senseless fairytales, believing that they somehow shielded themselves from reality in the imaginary world of myth. The truth is that all the Inklings were men of war. WWI slaughtered one-fifth of all Oxford students who were called to serve. All the Inklings were "comrades

---

76 Peter Jackson, *The Lord of the Rings: The Fellowship of the Ring* (New Line Cinema and WingNut Film, 2001).

77 Matthew 26:39.

78 J. R. R. Tolkien, *The Fellowship Of the Ring: Being the First Part of The Lord Of the Rings* (George Allen & Unwin, July 29, 1954).

who had been touched by war, who viewed life through the lens of war yet who looked for hope and found it in fellowship."[79]

We all need fortifications enriched by nurturing relationships to help protect us and encourage us during life's struggles, as well as sharing moments of happiness and accomplishments. We can learn from the hope the Inklings found in fellowship. I would add to Gandolf's charge that not only in such times must you decide what to do, but you must also choose with whom to do it. Choose and nurture your Allies wisely.

Summary

1. We are all consciously and subconsciously influenced by the people and environments surrounding us. You can manipulate the odds that these people play a positive role in your story by intentionally selecting those with whom you spend the most time. Reciprocally ask yourself, "Who do I need to become in order to be a better, more positive influence on the people I care about?"

2. People serve six broad roles in assisting your growth: Supporters, Masterminds, Mentors, Coaches, Professors, Professor Coaches. Which do you think will best propel your progress? What role can you play in shortcutting somebody else's growth?

3. Leaders throughout history have used mastermind groups as a means to constructively contribute to the lives of others as well as receive encouragement and direction for themselves. How can you harness the power of a mastermind to help you? How can you serve others by playing a leadership role in a mastermind?

---

79 Philip Zaleski and Carol Zaleski, *The Fellowship: The Literary Lives of the Inklings* (Farrar, Straus, and Giroux, 2015).

4. In what other types of positive group alliances can you become involved: service clubs, social clubs, faith-based small groups, twelve-step groups or therapy groups? How can you become a service to others through your participation?

5. Developing and maintaining healthy relationships is not a passive process and often requires us to lean into the discomfort and fear of changing familiar ways of relating. How many of the top ten tools do you naturally use? Which ones do you find the most difficult to adopt? The health of your relationships is dependent on the degree to which you are willing to do the uncomfortable.

As you complete this chapter, you may feel a little overwhelmed and unsure about how to incorporate and apply what you have learned from the first seven chapters in a meaningful and unified way. Robert McKee's advice to aspiring writers is especially apropos now. McKee recommended that in order to write a story that is believable and void of cliché, a writer must first dedicate time to developmental research. During this time a writer discovers the rich details of their characters' lives, values, strengths, struggles, emotions, and thoughts, as well as the important people and environments that surround them. The next common mistake McKee sees is that inexperienced writers often begin writing without outlining their story. According to McKee, the outline aims the trajectory of the story, defines its purpose and ensures that it comes to a sound conclusion.

In the next chapter you will learn a method to effectively outline, **Aim**, the story of your future self.

CHAPTER 7

Aim — Create Direction and A Plan for Your Life

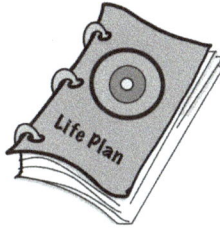

ARRIVAL GATE 1A: Adversity

DEPARTURE GATE 6A: Awareness, Attenuation, Assets, Allies, Aim, Action

Boarding Pass	Empowered Self-Care	Boarding Pass
Username: _____	**First Class**	← ✈ Departures
Destination: Beautiful Life	Current Location: Reality	
Arrival: **Gate 1A** (Adversity)		✈ **6A**
Departure: **Gate 6A** (Awareness, Attenuation, Assets, Allies, Aim, Action)		Gate

Most people think: planning is too restrictive and freedom is found in living for the moment.

The truth is: lack of planning limits our options and often chains us to unfavorable outcomes. Much of what is meaningful and fulfilling is acquired through intentional planning and diligent work.

"For it is better to Aim at one great task and complete it acceptably and with Honor, than to split your Aims into a dozen different Aims and win in none."[80]

"Aim at heaven and you will get earth thrown in. Aim at earth and you get neither."[81]

"What you aim at determines what you see."[82]

Amelia Earhart's Story

After becoming the first woman to cross the Atlantic Ocean by air and the first person to fly from Hawaii to the continental US, Amelia Earhart was thrust into stardom. Everybody wanted to see her, hear her speak and read about her daring adventures. She personified humanity's dream of shedding gravity's heavy hand and soaring on the waves of the wind.

The gifts that shaped her destiny, her independent nature and logical intellect, began to reveal themselves in the stories of her childhood. One of Amelia's elementary teachers reported that she, "Deduces the correct answers to complex arithmetic problems, but hates to put down the steps by which she arrived at the results."[83]

80 George Matthew Adams, *You Can: Road To Success* (George Matthew Adams, December 3, 2019).

81 C. S. Lewis, *The Joyful Christian: 127 Readings* (B & H Pub Group, April 1, 2000).

82 Jordan Peterson, *12 Rules of Life: An Antidote to Chaos* (Random House Canada, January 23, 2018).

83 Elgen M. Long and Marie K. Long, *Amelia Earhart: The Mystery Solved* (Simon and Schuster, 1999).

While in high school, Amelia's father moved the family six times in an effort to secure work. Deprived of time to nurture deep relationships, her strong natural tendency toward independence developed into a philosophy of living for the day. Amelia's sister said, "There was little room for nostalgia in AE's (Amelia Earhart's) character. She believed in living each day to the utmost, without wasting time in futile regrets over severed friendships or neglected opportunities."[84]

In 1917, Amelia's life changed forever. She met an officer in the Royal Canadian Flying Corps who invited her to the airfield to watch the pilots train. In her book *20 Hrs., 40 Min.*, Amelia wrote, "I remember well that when the snow blown back by the propellers stung my face, I felt the first urge to fly. I tried to get permission to go up, but the rules forbade [...] I have even forgotten the names of the men I knew then. But the memory of the planes remains clearly, and the sense of the inevitability of flying."[85]

Five years later, just little over a year and a half from her first flying lesson, on October 22, 1922, Amelia set a world record, becoming the first female pilot to fly at an altitude of 14,000 feet. On May 15, 1923, Amelia became the sixteenth female in the United States to be issued a formal pilot's license.

In 1928, Amelia received a call from publisher George Palmer Putnam that would catapult her life into the public eye. He invited her to be a passenger on the now famous "Friendship Flight," making her the first woman to fly across the Atlantic. Now in her early thirties, Amelia was exposed to the life of the rich and famous. Opportunity, excitement and adventure created an intoxicating elixir. Amelia's public schedule increasingly consumed more of her time, leaving less

---

84   Elgen M. Long and Marie K. Long, *Amelia Earhart: The Mystery Solved* (Simon and Schuster, 1999),

85   Amelia Earhart, *20 Min. 40 Hrs: Our Flight In The Friendship* (Martino Fine Books, August 28, 2014).

energy to maintain her flying skills and learn new emerging radio navigational and communication technologies.

In *Amelia Earhart: The Mystery Solved*, author Marie Long wrote, "She [Amelia] had learned early on the first commandment of the publicist: fame requires frequent public activity to keep your name in the news."[86] Not only did it require frequent activity, but as the public became numb to the novelty of aviation, she pushed herself to perform more spectacular flights. Caught in an escalating spiral of performing more dramatic and daring flights to maintain her lifestyle, Amelia pushed the envelope of safety.

Hoping for one last grand publicity stunt, Amelia proposed flying around the world. As opposed to others who had circumnavigated the earth using a northern route that limited time over water, Amelia wanted to fly as close to the equator as possible, or as she liked to say, "As near its waistline as could be."[87] Technology did not exist at the time, however, to fly nonstop across the vast expanses of the Pacific Ocean.

She had already flown the stretch from California to Hawaii once before, but she started in Hawaii and flew to California. It didn't take great navigational skills to hit the western coast of North America, but now she was proposing to start in California and fly westerly. Finding Hawaii would be difficult enough, but what then? Her solution was to land and refuel on Howland Island, a tiny island measuring 1.6 miles long x 0.6 miles wide, some 2,000 miles from any other significant land mass. She bet her life on finding a speck in the middle of the Pacific Ocean.

On March 17, 1937, Amelia began her first attempt to circumnavigate the world departing from Oakland, California bound for

---

86 Elgen M. Long and Marie K. Long, *Amelia Earhart: The Mystery Solved* (Simon and Schuster, 1999).

87 *Amelia Earhart: A Life From Beginning To End* (Hourly History, July 29, 2019).

Honolulu, Hawaii. During that initial leg, her plane developed mechanical problems, but she and the crew landed safely. The problems were more severe than she initially thought, delaying her departure. Two days later, the repairs were finally completed, and on the morning of March 20, 1937, Amelia was set to leave for Howland. With Amelia at the controls and no co-pilot in the right seat, for fear she would not be given full credit for the flight, the plane veered across the runway on takeoff and the propellers smashed into the pavement. Amelia's Lockheed Electra sustained massive damage, indefinitely delaying her circumnavigation. The cause of the crash was never clearly determined.

With huge international logistical hurdles to renegotiate, massive repair costs mounting, cash reserves dwindling, and a publicity nightmare to contend with, you can understand how Amelia could have felt overwhelmed. It was in this setting that Amelia made what turned out to be four fatal decisions. First, she did not rehire her chief radio navigation and communications expert, Harry Manning, even though she had not mastered the equipment herself. Second, she removed the long trailing wire antenna that extended her radio navigation and communication range. Third, she did not rehire Paul Mantz who served as her technical advisor, co-pilot and general assistant. And finally, she decided to reverse the direction of the trip. By doing this, she postponed the longest and riskiest legs, across the Pacific, to a time when she would be most exhausted.

Fred Noonan, the only person to accompany her on her second circumnavigation attempt, was suspected to have a drinking problem and, while an expert in celestial navigation, was much less knowledgeable about the new radio navigation and communications equipment installed in her plane.

On May 20, 1937, Amelia again departed Oakland, California, but this time she flew east-bound, marking the start of her second circumnavigation attempt. After flying to Miami, South America,

Africa, India, and Australia, and having flown over 22,000 miles, Amelia landed in the city of Lae, Papua New Guinea. This served as the final staging point for her legs across the Pacific. Drinking more heavily, Fred Noonan had become a liability over the course of the prior weeks. The decision not to rehire Paul Mantz and Henry Manning was now an obvious mistake. With nobody to help share the workload and manage the flights, Earhart was ill and exhausted. Instead of stopping, resting and letting herself heal, she pressed on. When she needed every ounce of cognitive skill, she abandoned reason and decided to continue toward the minuscule Howland Island 2,600 miles to the east, in the middle of the Pacific Ocean.

On July 2, 1937, midnight GMT, Amelia Earhart and Fred Noonan took off from Lae Airfield, hoping to reach the island in an estimated time of eighteen hours. Having removed her antenna, never learning Morse code and not fully understanding how to use her radio navigational and communication equipment, Earhart put all her trust in the abilities of the alcohol-impaired Fred Noonan and his celestial navigation skills. They might have made it in clear weather, but their flight path was littered with clouds. Noonan likely had a difficult time getting accurate readings. Even in the best of circumstances, the window of error with celestial navigation is plus/minus 10 percent. That may not sound like much, but stretched over 2,600 miles, it made all the difference in the world when trying to locate a tiny island.

Her risk-taking had paid off in the past. With the Friendship Flight that had catapulted her to fame they had also flown into cloudy conditions with little fuel reserve, and depended only on celestial navigation. The big difference was that then they were trying to locate Europe, much like her flight from Hawaii to California—not a difficult process if they just stayed on a single compass reading.

Earhart and Noonan probably came within fifty miles of the island. The *Itasca*, a US navy ship, was anchored off Howland Island to help guide them. They could hear Earhart's verbal communications, but she could not hear them. She could pick up the radio navigation signal the *Itasca* was sending, but she couldn't determine the direction from which it was coming. Fred Noonan was of no help in either case. If they had had enough fuel reserve, they could have run a search pattern and found the island. Another poor planning error, failing to wait for more favorable headwinds, depleted most of their fuel reserves.

As we know, Earhart never made it. Running desperately low on fuel, at 8:43 a.m. on July 2, 1937, Amelia spoke her last recorded words, "We are running North and South." Most likely, they were lost and running a search pattern for the island. Nobody knows what happened after that, but she likely ditched the plane in the ocean where it sank some 18,000 feet below. Search efforts ended on July 19, 1937. America's national treasure was lost forever.

Aviation's Lessons for the Non-Pilot

Earhart's story is sad because it was preventable. In hindsight, it's easy to see the series of circumstances and poor decisions that lead to her ill-fated flight. Aviation has learned from her tragedy and many others like it. Appropriate planning and managing cockpit workload is key to preventing similar crashes. As we have already discussed, we all have limited mental resources and once those resources are used, we default to less accurate and more automatic mental shortcuts. In our daily routine, these shortcuts may simply foster and maintain unwanted unhealthy habits, but in the cockpit the mistakes they induce can kill.

Most crashes are the result of human error, and occur during high workload environments. To help promote efficient critical thinking during these times, the Federal Aviation Administration (FAA) has established several rules of operation for commercial flights:

1. They must be crewed by two pilots.

2. Crews must maintain a "sterile cockpit" during periods of high workload. Crew members are prohibited from performing non-essential duties or activities while the aircraft is involved in taxi, takeoff, landing, and all other flight operations conducted below 10,000 feet.

3. A flight plan must be filed, and include among other things the route, destination, estimated time, and the amount of fuel on board.

We can learn from these recommendations. You may not be attempting a groundbreaking circumnavigation of the world or planning to pilot a commercial flight, but all of us are piloting our own journeys riddled with unforeseen stress-inducing obstacles.

Three Rules for Piloting Your Life:

1. Include trusted friends in your decision-making. Sometimes all you need is another perspective. Phone an Ally.

2. Limit distractions and focus on the most important issues. Prioritize tasks.

3. Develop a thorough plan for your journey. Write a Life Plan.

Common Mental Energy Resource

In the 1960s Walter Mischel performed the now famous Marshmallow Test with preschoolers at Stanford University's Bing Nursery. Mischel allowed children to pick their favorite snack from a large selection of marshmallows, cookies, pretzels, mints, and chocolates. He then presented the preschoolers with a choice: receive one of your favorite snacks now, or receive two if you can wait for twenty minutes alone.

If they chose to wait, he placed their favorite snack on a table and had the child sit on a chair in front of it. They were instructed to stay seated. If they left the chair or ate even one bite of the snack before the allotted time, the experiment was over. The proctor then left the room while Mischel and his team watched the children through a one-way mirror. For one set of children, the temptation of immediate gratification was too great, and they settled for the expedient—but smaller—reward. The other group, given the exact same conditions, resisted and for their efforts received the greater reward.

Mischel and his team tracked these children into adulthood and discovered that the differences they noted at ages four and five followed them throughout their life. The children who were able to delay gratification went on to achieve higher SAT scores, developed a better sense of self-worth, maintained a lower body mass index, cultivated better relationships, and achieved higher incomes.

Unfortunately, his work on self-control went largely unrecognized for decades. Throughout the 1960s and into the 1980s, child psychologists continued to ignore Mischel's work and encouraged parents and educators to nurture positive self-esteem in lieu of self-control.

It was not until twenty years later in the 1980s that Roy Baumeister reluctantly stumbled across Mischel's work and the concept of self-control and willpower. Baumeister reports that he was deeply entrenched in the popular self-esteem philosophy, but evidence for self-esteem began to reveal disappointing results. One such study showed that despite exceptionally high self-confidence in their scholastic abilities, US students were falling far below Korean and Japanese students who had far less self-esteem. Encouraging self-esteem in the face of poor performance undermines long-term self-control and success.[88]

Baumeister returned to Mischel's work to better understand why some children were better at delayed gratification. He noticed that instant-gratifiers and delayed-gratifiers used different strategies. Instant-gratifiers stared at the treats, sniffed them, held them, and even licked them. Eventually temptation overwhelmed them. The delayed-gratifiers, on the other hand, covered the cookies, looked in the opposite direction, sang songs, and told themselves stories until the proctor returned. In essence, they distracted themselves. The delayed-gratifiers did not necessarily have more self-control; they just used their self-control differently. They conserved their self-control by limiting temptation. He hypothesized that self-control exists in a limited supply and must be used efficiently.

After performing a series of experiments, Baumeister and his postdoctoral students concluded that both resisting temptation and decision-making use a common consumable mental energy resource. In 2011, Jonathan Levav from Columbia University and Shai Danziger from Ben-Gurion University reviewed 1,112 parole cases of eight Jewish-Israeli judges. They proposed that if making serial decisions is linked to a limited depletable common mental energy resource (CMER), then the quality of the judges' decisions would degrade as their CMER level drops.

Each studied judge deliberated 14-35 cases daily and each deliberation lasted for approximately six minutes. During the day, the judges took two breaks: a mid-morning break that lasted approximately forty minutes, and an early afternoon lunch break that lasted

---

88   Ina V. S. Mullis et al., Chapter 4: Student's Backgrounds and Attitudes Towards Mathematics. TIMSS 1999 International Mathematics Report: Findings from IEA's Repeat of the Third International Mathematics and Science Study at the Eighth Grade (Chestnut Hill, MA: International Study Center, Boston College, Lynch School of Education, 2000).

for approximately one hour. These two breaks divided their day into three working sessions. At the beginning of the day, parole rates were around 65 percent but by the end of the morning work session, the rate dropped to nearly zero. After the morning break, parole rates returned to approximately 65 percent and dropped again to about 15 percent toward the end. After the lunch break, parole rates once again increased back to 65 percent and by the end of the day they again dropped to nearly zero (see Figure 7.1)

When the Surface Brain's capacity to think rationally becomes overwhelmed, the brain simplifies its thinking processes. It diverts decision-making to the Deep Brain's more automatic patterns or shortcuts. Like pilots who make more mistakes when their workload increases, the intense workload and time constraints of the judges' schedule accentuated the emotional burden and the tendency to default to automatic thinking.

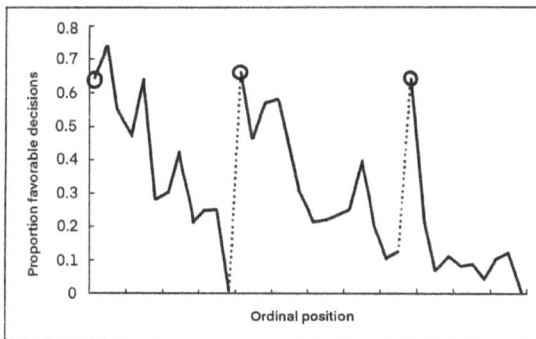

Proportion of rulings in favor of the prisoners by ordinal position. Circled points indicate the first decision in each of the three decision sessions; tick marks on x axis denote every third case; dotted line denotes food break. Because unequal session lengths resulted in a low number of cases for some of the later ordinal positions, the graph is based on the first 95% of the date from each session.

(FIGURE 7.1)[89]

---

89 Shai Danziger, Jonathan Levav, and Liora Avnaim-Pesso, *Extraneous Factors in Judicial Decisions* (Proceedings of the National Academy of Sciences, April 26, 2011).

The judges subconsciously and automatically simplified the decision-making process by accepting the status quo, i.e. leaving the prisoner in jail. The safest thing for society is to leave a potentially dangerous criminal in jail. If unsure, the judges' conscience was eased by accepting this default. Even the most conscientious judges were not immune to the effects of CMER depletion and automatic thinking. You and I are not immune to it either.

Another interesting finding in this study is that while CMER is depletable, it is also renewable. After short breaks, the judges' leniency returned to baseline. Possible replenishing factors during the breaks include glucose consumption (food intake), rest and improved mood. If you need to make a series of important decisions, give yourself enough time and take several replenishing breaks.

Numerous similar studies have discovered that several different types of mental processes are powered by this same depletable CMER:

1. Thought Control: Long periods of decision-making, calculating or planning use and deplete CMER.

2. Emotional Control: When in a bad mood or in constant pain, we use CMER to regulate our emotions.

3. Impulse Control: Environments rich in temptations consume CMER, leaving us vulnerable to making poor decisions.

4. Performance Control: Focusing on a task while regulating the balance between accuracy and speed, managing time and persevering depletes CMER.

As any one of these processes depletes your CMER, the other processes suffer by defaulting to automatic thinking processes. Because self-control is an aggregate of thought control, emotional control, impulse control, and performance control, it is vulnerable to depletion as CMER levels drop. If self-control diminishes as your CMER levels drop, then conserving CMER is a key ingredient in building and sustaining healthy habits, as well as making positive change.

Write Your Life Plan

(An outline for writing your Life Plan can be found in the Summary at the end of the chapter.)

Following the learned experience of pilots who write a flight plan and successful writers who outline their stories, we are going to embark on outlining your life's trajectory by writing a Life Plan in an effort to maximize your limited capacity of CMER.

Adam Brantley, one of my previous executive coaches, gave me this advice, "When you have a clear and compelling vision in place for your personal life, it directly bleeds into everything else you do. It allows you to engage much more vibrantly. It doesn't mean that you will do everything perfectly. Your life plan allows you to put a stake in the ground, mark where you are today, your current reality, clearly see where you want to go, who is it that you want to be, what's the legacy you want to leave, and then answer the question, 'How am I going to bridge that gap?'"

As you start to create your Life Plan, keep these tips in mind:

1. Time to Think

Limit distraction. Set aside time to devote solely to this task. Make this time a priority. Schedule a weekend for yourself, preferably not at home or work. Go to a beautiful, inspiring place where you can concentrate on this singular task. Turn your digital devices off, especially your cellphone. Limit all distractions and commit to completing at least a rough draft of your Life Plan.

Your Life Plan will never be complete. You will learn much about yourself as you start living more intentionally. Unforeseen opportunities will also appear if you are paying attention. These opportunities will dictate changes in your Life Plan, so it is important to revisit it at least yearly.

Action step

Open your calendar and decide when you will do this. Place it on your schedule. Tell those who need to know—family, friends, coworkers—that you will be unavailable during this time.

2. Aged Portrait

One insurance company tried a novel approach to encourage their customers to save more for retirement. They hypothesized that one of the reasons people don't save enough for retirement is they can't see themselves as an older person who will need the funds. To help make the older version of themselves appear more real, they took a picture of their clients and ran it through an aging program. Those who reviewed their retirement goals daily while viewing the aged picture saved twice as much.

Download an app like "Aging Booth" or "FaceLab" and age a picture of yourself. The picture to the left is a photo of me the weekend I wrote my first Life Plan (Image 7.2). The picture to the right is the picture I created and reviewed as I wrote my Life Plan.

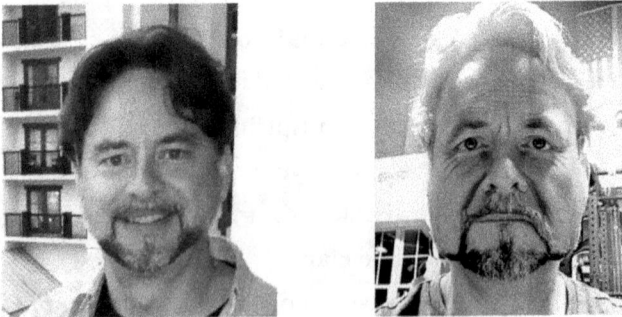

(IMAGE 7.2)

I framed the picture and set it on my desk so I couldn't avoid it as I wrote my Life Plan. Surprisingly, it affected me emotionally more than I had anticipated.

Action Step

Download a photo aging app and age your picture. Print a copy so you can view it as you write your Life Plan.

3. A Better Version of You

What does a better version of yourself look like? Focus on becoming more of you, and not someone different. You were uniquely and completely gifted from the beginning with all the talents you need to become who you were designed to be. While you already possess a complete set of raw talents, within them are the skills you need to develop. What are they?

Remember that perfection is not the goal. Aim for steady progress and improvement. Setbacks are a necessary part of your journey. Much of what makes life meaningful is found in moments of discomfort. Envision a life capable of adapting to the ebbs and flows.

With your aged picture in hand, look into your eyes. Imagine that aged version of you at the end of your life surrounded by the people you care about most. Picture yourself reminiscing about a life well lived. Relive all your exciting adventures and memorable moments. Feel the warmth of an overwhelming love. As you witness this, the scene suddenly freezes and your aged self locks eyes at you and calls you to an extraordinary adventure. They urge you to stop wasting time, to seize the moment, to live a life of significance, and to become more of the person you are called to be.

What is your aged self saying to you? To what journey are you being called? For what purpose?

The book of Exodus tells the story of how Moses was called to the top of Mount Sinai where he witnessed God write the Ten Commandments for the nation of Israel. You probably haven't had a similar experience, but if your aged self could encourage you to follow ten principles of wellbeing or ten core virtues, what would they be?

Happiness researcher Dr. Michael Frisch and his team at Baylor University composed an exhaustive list of what he calls Tenets of Contentment. Consistent with the story of Moses, Frisch recognized that the quality of peoples' lives directly correlates with the tenets by which they live. You can review a copy of Frisch's Tenets of Contentment[90] at www.DrYou.org/resources.

As we have already discussed, not all values are virtuous and thus not all values lead to contentment and wellbeing. Given the limit of our own life span and cognitive capacity it makes sense to me to learn from the pool of scientific literature, examples in history and the sacred teachings of those that have contemplated these concepts for millennia.

Many argue that one of the major historical contributions western civilization has made to humanity has been the codification of a common universal value system based on the Biblical text. Some even argue that it is because of this common value system that western civilization has seen such success. Even if you do not accept the authenticity of the Biblical text, it is hard to deny the impact it has had on the west's historical values. Take for example these ten virtues. Do they sound familiar?

1. Aim at the highest possible good, true and beautiful imaginable.

2. Don't confuse a surrogate of truth with actual truth.

---

90   Michael B. Frisch, *Quality of Life Therapy: Applying a Life Satisfaction Approach to Positive Psychology and Cognitive Therapy* (John Wiley & Sons, 2006).

3. Don't belittle the highest good even in small ways, for as you do in small ways so will you do in larger more important ways.

4. Set aside time to contemplate and show gratitude for all that is truly important.

5. Show respect to those who have made sacrifices for you.

6. Honor the lives of others both by your actions and in your thoughts.

7. Commit to the people you love, especially your spouse.

8. Respect the labor of honest, hard-working individuals.

9. Don't speak words that maliciously harm others.

10. Seek comprehensive solutions, as simple answers foster envy and resentment.

We see these values as virtuous in part because of our common Judeo-Christian history. These are simple rephases of the Old Testament Ten Commandments.

Aiming is fundamentally a proposition of value. As we prioritize one envisioned outcome, we de-emphasize another we have deemed less important. How can you ensure your visions are consistent with values that propagate beautiful living?

What are your top ten tenets, values or principles of wellbeing? How can you use history, science and sacred teachings to verify that your perceived values are not leading you down unhealthy paths?

As you think about what you could be, what your aged self encourages you to become, make sure to incorporate these top tenets or virtues into your story. Close your eyes and envision all the small details. Write down what you want the better version of yourself to look like. Your vision needs to excite you. This is your vision— it doesn't belong to your spouse, your pastor, priest or rabbi, your parents or your friends. What are the things you have always wanted to do, but have been afraid to express or pursue?

Action Step

    a. At the top of a piece of paper write, "The Vision," "Better Version of Me," "The Dream," or whatever title captures your imagination.

    b. Below that write, "Ten Principles of Wellbeing" and list your top ten principles for living or top ten ideal virtues.

    c. Below your ten principles/virtues, write three or four paragraphs that describe the person you want to become. What do you want those you care about and will be with you at the end of your life to say? How does this vision propagate or is at least consistent with your top principles of wellbeing or virtues? Some think in terms of writing their own obituary. What do you want that to say?

    d. Write two or three sentences that summarize your overall vision. Think of this as a personal "mission statement."

You can download a copy of the "Better Version of You" template at www. DrYou.org/resources.

BETTER VERSION OF YOU

Title:

Ten Principles of Wellbeing:
1.
2.
3.
4.
5.
6.
7.
8.
9.
10.

The Vision:

(FIGURE 7.3 — 1 OF 2)

Title:

The Vision (continued):

Mission Statement:

(FIGURE 7.3 — 2 OF 2)

4. Life Domains

In the Introduction, I presented the analogy of life as a rope composed of different interwoven strands. Each of these strands represents a domain of your life. Together these domains function as a single unit. Your life's overall strength, therefore, depends on the strength of each individual domain.

Not all life domains are equal. Investing in some, such as money, fame, power, and pleasure increase happiness—but only briefly. Social scientists call this transient feeling hedonic adaptation. With hedonic adaptation, your mood varies from its baseline, but it eventually returns to normal. For example, if somebody were to give you a new car, you would feel happy for a period of time. Eventually, however, your mood would drift back to your baseline. This is not necessarily a bad thing. What would happen if you ate a splendid meal and said, "Wow this was a wonderful meal. I am so perpetually satisfied that I don't think I'll ever eat again." Hedonic adaptation is one of the driving forces that keeps us motivated to provide for ourselves and others.

Hedonic adaptation also helps you adjust to unhappy circumstances. If your spouse decides to leave you for another person, you will experience turmoil. As time passes, however, hedonic adaptation pulls your mood back up to your previous happier baseline.

The term "subjective wellbeing" is a more meaningful one than "happiness." Happiness can mean so many things that it fundamentally means nothing at all. For many, living a life of happiness implies pursuing a state of continuous bliss. Continuous bliss is impossible and, more importantly, it devalues the role of discomfort in growth and contentment. Subjective wellbeing, on the other hand, is a more comprehensive term that describes a life capable of experiencing contentment and growth in moments of pleasure and pain.

The problem, therefore, is two-fold:

1. The pursuit of a simple transient positive affect, "happiness," instead of creating a more complex and nuanced state of "subjective wellbeing."

2. Investing too heavily in quickly adapting life domains (money, pleasure, power, and fame) versus more stable life domains (faith, family, friends, and work.)

My list of Life Domains includes physical health, spiritual health, cognitive health, emotional health, spouse, children, family, friends, career, finances, and hobbies.

You may want to make a different list or add other domains. Consider some of these:

- Values/spiritual health/identity/goals/faith

- Self-compassion/self-esteem/emotional health

- Physical health

- Relationships/love/affection/inclusion/family/friends

- Career/work/retirement

- Play/recovery/hobbies/recreation

- Helping/altruism

- Learning/mastery

- Creativity/achievement/tasks bigger than yourself

- Finances/money/standard of living/sustenance

- Surroundings/community

What am I doing today to progress the dream?

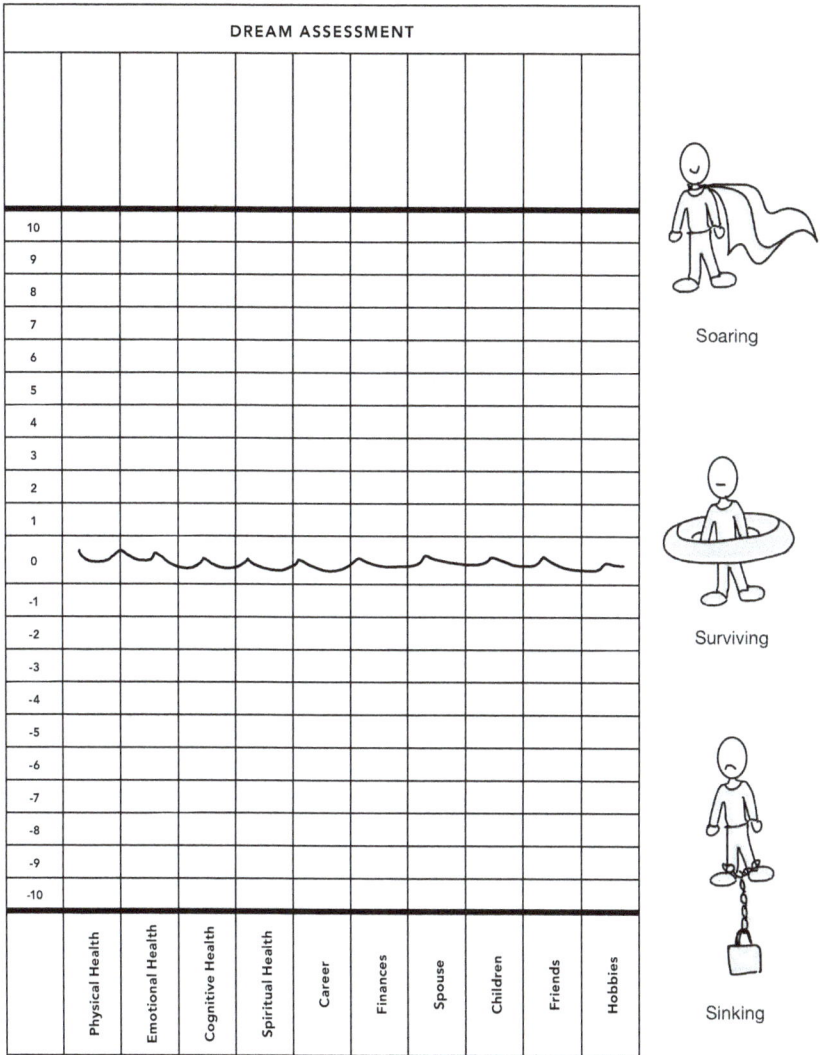

(FIGURE 7.4)

Don't forget time for recovery. Recovery comes in two forms:

1. Rest, the passive form.

2. Recreation, the active form.

As we learned from the Israeli judges, we all need time to replenish our mental and physical resources. Intentionally build time into your schedule for both forms of recovery. For me, this falls under my "Hobbies" Domain.

Action Step

What are your most important or crucial top ten life domains? List them along the bottom of the Dream Assessment Tool above (Figure 7.4.) You can download a separate copy of the dream assessment tool, or you can download it as a part of the Life Plan template at www. DrYou.org/resources. Maybe you think only five domains are crucial for your growth. That's fine. List the ones that are important to you. Limit the number of domains to ten, however, otherwise they become too overwhelming to work with.

5. Destination

Now that you have a clear idea of your overall mission and the most important domains involved in it, let's create a compelling vision for each domain.

Look back at your aged picture. I know it still sounds hokey, but stare into your aged self's eyes again. Transport yourself into the future and listen to what that version of yourself would tell your current self. What lessons did you learn along the way? What paths/detours would you avoid? What opportunities would you pursue that you were afraid to take?

Create a destination that excites you and is meaningful to you. This is not a time to be shy or think small. Dream big. Author Jim Collins suggests you create a Big Hairy Audacious Goal or BHAG (pronounced "Bee hag.") We'll get to small practical goals under Action Steps. That's not what I want you to do now. I want you to aim for the stars. If everything were to go perfectly, what would each domain look like at the end of your life? Don't worry if it isn't practical, and don't worry about what anybody else thinks. Nobody will see this unless you decide to show them.

What are the secret desires you have been afraid to share with anybody? Write them down now. Are you excited yet? If not, keep digging.

Remember to keep in mind your Giftedness, your Principles of Wellbeing, and your Purpose.

Action Steps

    a. For each domain, take a separate sheet of paper and write the name of the Life Domain at the top.

    b. Write two to three paragraphs that describe your vision for each domain. Think of this as the destination you are trying to reach.

LIFE DOMAIN:
1
2
3

6. *Note the Gap*

As you may have noticed, you are creating a story about becoming a better version of yourself. As such, let's revisit Robert McKee's instructions for writing compelling stories. He contends that good stories follow a common structure: inciting event, progressive complication, crisis, climax, resolution. This structure helps successful writers create an emotional, tension-filled gap that clearly delineates the results the protagonist desires (destination) and the results he actually achieves (reality.) According to McKee, this gap is the power that drives the story, tension that can only be resolved by completing the story. Without the tension, the story fizzles.

You also want to create clear gaps to compel you to complete your story. Similar to those of the protagonist, your gaps are the differences between where you are currently (reality) and what you want to achieve (destination.)

Go back to your Dream Assessment Tool (Figure 7.4.) Above each domain column, write one or two words that will remind you of the destination you are trying to reach, your BHAG for each domain.

Now close your eyes and envision how well you are doing in each domain. Concentrate on one at a time. Envision the goal, then subjectively rank how well you are achieving it on a scale from -10 to +10. A -10 is failing miserably. You feel like you are drowning and being pulled under into the abyss. A 0 is equivalent to floating in the middle of the Pacific. You aren't drowning, but you're certainly not thriving. You are just surviving. A +10 is equivalent to hitting it out of the ballpark. You are soaring! Place a checkmark on the Dream Assessment Tool that denotes that ranking. Allow yourself to feel the tension and discomfort as you clearly note the gap between your current reality and your desired destination.

Some social scientists suggest that people are happy to the extent they see a favorable comparison between their reality and their destination. In my experience, people see subjective wellbeing not only when their reality and their vision match, but also when they create a clear and compelling plan to bridge the gap and then begin taking concrete steps to close it. Subjective Wellbeing, therefore, does not require you to achieve your ultimate destination, your BHAG. It is contingent, however, on you actively pursuing a plan to close the gap. It is all about the journey.

Benjamin Franklin is famous for his book of virtues. He carried an ivory notebook in which he had drawn a chart with thirteen virtues listed in individual roles similar to Figure 7.5. To the right he drew seven columns, one for each day of the week. Each week, he would concentrate on trying to master one of the virtues. At the end of each day, he would place a black "spot" in the corresponding block for that virtue and day of the week if he had violated any virtues. The goal was to live an entire week without placing a single black spot on the chart.

VIRTUE DIARY

	Sun	Wed	Tues	Wed	Thurs	Fri	Sat
Temperance							
Silence							
Order							
Resolution							
Frugality							
Industry							
Sincerity							
Justice							
Moderation							
Cleanliness							
Tranquility							
Chastity							
Humility							

(FIGURE 7.5)

The task was more difficult than Franklin initially anticipated. He said, "I was surpris'd to find myself so much fuller of faults than I had imagined."[91]

He conceded that he never accomplished the task of living a completely virtuous life, but admitted, "On the whole, tho' I never arrived at the perfection I had been so ambitious of obtaining, but fell far short of it, yet I was, by the endeavor a better and happier man than I otherwise should have been if I had not attempted it."[92]

Action Steps

a. On your Dream Assessment Chart write one or two words that summarize your goals at the top of each domain column.

b. Subjectively rank how well you are doing in each domain.

c. Note the gap between your vision and your current reality. Embrace the discomfort and use it to motivate you to change.

8. Purpose

In the summer of 2018, my wife Sara and I spent a couple of weeks in the Serengeti photographing lions, elephants, giraffes, wildebeest, zebras, hippos, and cheetahs. Actually, Sara photographed while I tagged along. It was an amazing experience, and our clinic is filled with Sara's beautiful work. As we roamed the Serengeti, I visited some of the local Maasai people with our guides. Our basic struggles were similar: How do we provide for our families? How can we most effectively educate our children? How can we protect the people we love? How do we do something meaningful? Where do we find significance?

---

91 Benjamin Franklin, *Benjamin Franklin's Book of Virtues* (Applewood Books, September 27, 2016).

92 Benjamin Franklin, *Benjamin Franklin's Book of Virtues* (Applewood Books, September 27, 2016).

They seemed to be excelling at these most basic yet important tasks without the benefit of a big house, pool, cars, expensive vacations, and fancy clothes. In reality, my house is neither big nor fancy, and my clothes are certainly not chic. In their eyes, however, I was wealthy.

Life there was slower. The people spent a significant amount of their time socializing with each other, not through texts, Facebook or other online media, but in person. They danced, sang, joked, and laughed together in person. By default, their lives were simpler, but relationship-centric and purpose-driven—a natural recipe for subjective wellbeing.

Life may have been slower, but that didn't mean it was devoid of work. Abject poverty is a tragedy and causes much suffering. Those who were most "successful," like our guides, didn't merely sit around and visit with friends all day. They didn't passively wait for their fate to change. They worked hard to provide a better life for themselves and their families. Our guides were intelligent, educated men. They didn't have master's degrees or doctorates, but they had spent a lifetime learning. They were walking encyclopedias of the local wildlife and fauna. Their work wasn't only about providing for their families; it was a sacred task. Part of that mission, their sacred task, was preserving the Serengeti by educating tourists like us.

In the Christian New Testament, the apostle Matthew shared this parable of Jesus:

> "Then he told them many things in parables, saying: 'A farmer went out to sow his seed. As he was scattering the seed, some fell along the path, and the birds came and ate it up. Some fell on rocky places, where it did not have much soil. It sprang up quickly, because the soil was shallow. But when the sun came up, the plants were scorched, and they withered because they had not root. Other seed fell among thorns, which grew up and choked the plants. Still other seed fell on good soil, where it pro-

duced a crop—a hundred, sixty or thirty times what was sown. Whoever has ears, let them hear."[93]

Ancient parables like this one are said to contain many layers of meaning, like an onion. One layer of this parable suggests that you can focus your efforts in many places. Some endeavors will produce temporary pleasures, but they quickly fade. With rich, fertile endeavors your results will not be exponentially better. Work for which you are uniquely designed with an emphasis on serving others is an example of fertile endeavors that yield results thirty, sixty or even 160 times more than others.

Pursuing endeavors that result in power, fortune and fame are not necessarily without purpose. The problem comes when the primary focus is this power, fortune or fame. You can build an external life full of wealth as long as you simultaneously pursue an internal life of purpose—and the two must be coherent with each other. If they are discordant, your life will be filled with angst.

Another way I like to think of Life Domains are as gears inside a machine. This machine represents my life and the work I am tasked to accomplish. Taped to my bathroom mirror is this picture (Figure 7.6.) It reminds me of the core principles for living well.

Simple images such as this are important because they communicate to your Deep Brain in a way words cannot.

My machine looks like something out of a children's story book. Like me, it's a little clunky, a bit odd and incomplete in many ways. It's not perfect either, as I am still a work in progress. Yours may look more like a beautiful Italian sports car or a Rolex watch. Whatever it looks like, I encourage you to draw your own version.

---

93 Matthew 13:3-9.

Note how each individual gear is a different size. This represents the relative importance we place on each domain during different seasons of life. Also, note that the gears' teeth vary in size and quantity. While we are all gifted with the basic resources to live a beautiful life, we must nurture and grow the appropriate skills and competencies for each domain. This is an intentional process that requires persistent work. The gear teeth represent those skills and competencies. In a life well lived, all domains/gears possess a full set of healthy teeth. In reality, we often emphasize the development of some life skills at the expense of others. What skills do you need to develop? Is one of your life domains inappropriately under- or overemphasized for this particular season of your life?

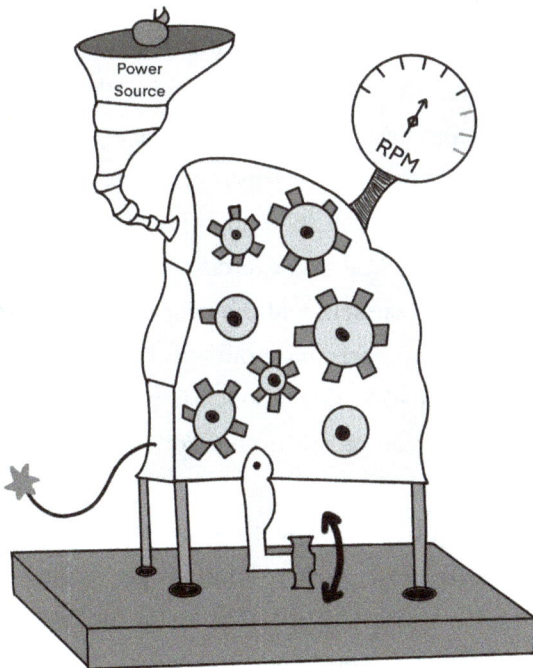

(FIGURE 7.6)

At the bottom, you can see an arm with a hammer head. This represents the work the machine was designed to do—your meaningful work. Your meaningful work is the practical application of your set of unique gifts or motivated abilities. Do you know what that work is? Are you consistently doing it?

The three legs are the pillars of human needs. Humans have nine basic needs. Each leg represents three:

Leg 1: Affection, inclusion and autonomy

Leg 2: Meaningful work, identity and security

Leg 3: Mastery, sustenance and recovery

Your life and its meaningful work is built on a foundation of meeting both your needs and others'. A healthy life requires both.

In the top left corner, there is a funnel to represent the power source. These are all the external factors that influence your thoughts, beliefs and behaviors. With what are you feeding or powering yourself? In a literal sense, this represents the food with which you power your body. Is your food nutritious and wholesome or is it toxic? It also represents how you exercise, the amount of rest you get or how you recharge yourself, and the people, systems, and environments with which you surround yourself. How empowering is the content you consume—TV, radio, podcasts, music? All these factors can either empower you or drain you. You get to decide; just don't leave them to chance.

In the upper right corner, there's a tachometer. In your car, the tachometer indicates how many revolutions per minute (RPMs) your engine rotates. It's a safety gauge. If you run the engine too fast or redline it, you can burn it up. As a part of my life machine, it reminds me to keep my activities in the optimal range. When you work outside this range, you risk burnout. Three factors help keep our work meaningful and sustain our motivation:

R: Relevant. Meaningful work must be relevant to you, nobody else.

P: Purposeful. Meaningful work is bigger than you, and therefore not only meets your needs, but also others' needs.

M: Movement. Meaningful work implies motion. If you aren't moving, you aren't making progress. Talking about meaningful work is not movement. Talking is spinning your wheels in place. You must take action.

Finally, you'll note something that looks like a tail extending to the bottom left. This is your life fuse. It was lit the moment you were born and will burn 24/7 until the moment you die. None of us knows how long our fuse initially was, and none of us knows how much fuse we have left. Make every moment count.

As you write the narrative for each of your Life Domains, how do each of these domains help you accomplish your sacred task, your purpose, your meaningful work? As an essential gear to produce your meaningful work, what must each of those areas look like? What skills and competencies must you develop in each? What are the fertile endeavors that will not only produce results, but exponential results?

Action Steps

a. Draw a picture that reminds you of your sacred task and your core principles of living well. If you don't like drawing, find a picture online or in a magazine that represents them. You're welcome to copy mine.

b. Place your drawing in a conspicuous place so it reminds you of the work you need to do. Also include a copy of your drawing/picture in your Life Plan.

c. How does each domain integrate into your sacred task? How can you incorporate your unique strengths into that process? For each domain write a few sentences under Purpose that clarifies and summarizes those ideas for you.

9. Allies

In the chapter on Allies, we discussed how external factors, especially people, can foster and encourage your growth. When designing your Life Plan, consider how to intentionally surround yourself with such Allies. Also think about people for whom you can be an encouraging ally. If you were to set up a mastermind or personal board of advisors to help inspire and keep you motivated, who would those people be?

People can serve as a positive influence whether they are dead or alive. Which historical figures inspire you? Commit to consuming more of their content or content about them. Include in your Life Plan some of their inspirational quotes. Memorize some of their most influential sayings. Keep a list of these in a diary or on notecards so you can easily review them. How can you continuously feed yourself with such positive content?

Be intentional about developing relationships. Life can get so busy that we lose focus on people. When was the last time you called a mentor to thank them? When was the last time you called a friend to meet for lunch with no agenda other than to invest in the relationship?

What news, media, podcasts, books, music, and TV programs do you need to intentionally consume? What do you need to jettison? Add that to your Life Plan. What you consume will influence your progress. Intentionally design an environment that promotes the proper mindset of success and embraces beliefs, habits and routines that help you accomplish your goals. Shun influences that hinder your progress.

Can you shape your physical environment to serve as a better positive Ally? My office and home are filled with visual reminders: a horse-and-rider statue, a life machine picture, photographs, a sand timer, rocks in a glass tube (each rock represents a week remaining in my life.) What visual reminders, inspirational images or works of art do you need to include in your physical environment?

Action Steps

a. Make a list of people you want to include in your personal board of advisors.

b. Consider starting your own mastermind group. Make a list of people you'd like to join it.

c. Make a list of thought leaders whose content you want to consume more of.

d. Find encouraging quotes from those thought leaders and include some of them in this section of your Life Plan. In what other places can you display their quotes to inspire you?

e. Make a list of other relationships you need to spend more time nurturing.

f. List ways you can arrange your physical environment to more effectively serve you. Make a list of visual reminders you want to include. Do you need to make the space more inviting by organizing it better or decluttering it? Do you need to beautify it in some way? List all your thoughts.

10. SMARTER steps

Grand goals, BHAGs and ultimate life destinations can be exciting, but they also can feel so out of reach that they overwhelm instead of inspire. The trick is to dream big while simultaneously creating smaller, practical steps that feel more achievable. Flight plans accomplish this for pilots. When pilots map out a flight plan, they locate their home airport and then their final destination. Often they don't simply fly straight from their starting point to their destination. Instead, with modern GPS units, they map out a series of waypoints that lead to their final destination. What waypoints do you need to link together to reach your end goal?

SMARTER Goals

The concept of SMART goals was developed by George Doran, Arthur Miller and James Cunningham in 1981. I heard a speaker at a conference talk about SMARTER goals, which is a twist on their original concept.

> **S: Specific.** Too many people write vague goals. Specific goals help clarify what success looks like. If you don't know this, how will you know you've reached it once you're there? Make sure your goals are process goals, not outcome goals. Outcome goals are your BHAG final destination goals. Process goals are the smaller, concrete action steps you take to reach your final destination. Let's use weight loss as an example. Good process goals would be to eat 4-5 servings of vegetables and walk for forty-five minutes a day. Process goals are directly within your power to achieve right now.

> **M: Measurable.** Make sure these steps can be quantified in concrete ways. For example, I am going to exercise for sixty minutes a day, walk 10,000 steps a day, read thirty pages a day or write 500-1,000 words a day.

> **A: Attainable.** These steps need to be realistic and easy to achieve. You want them to challenge you, but not overwhelm you. Remember the diagram of Flow. Mihaly Csikszentmihalyi suggests that a good goal should be just 10-20 percent beyond your current com-

petency. That is enough to challenge you, but not so much to discourage you.

R: Relevant. Your goals must be important to you. It doesn't matter what anybody else thinks or wants you to do.

T: Time-bound. Set a reasonable time limit to achieve your goal, then write it on a calendar. Projects expand to the amount of time we set aside to complete them. Goals do the same.

E: Exciting. Your goals should be compelling and motivating. Life is short. You might as well spend your life working on things that energize and excite you.

R: Recorded. Write them down. Goals not written are only wishes.

As you write your SMARTER goals, remember to ask yourself, "Who do I need to become in order to reach my destination?" It's not about just doing more things, but becoming more of who you were designed to be. There must be a shift in focus from external—the things you must do and circumstances you must change—to internal—what you must become. By doing this, you will automatically align your goals with your core values and with your natural giftedness.

Action Steps

For each domain, list the very next SMARTER step you need to accomplish to move you closer to your desired destination. You don't need to know all the steps that lead to your BHAG. All you need to know is the very next step. I have found that once I accomplish that step, the next step becomes clearer.

11. Obstacles

Part of you wants to make the changes necessary to grow, and part of you likes the status quo. The part of you that doesn't want to change may be afraid of losing a benefit that your current lifestyle is providing.

Take physical fitness. Part of you may want to get in better shape. This rational-thinking part recognizes all the long-term benefits. Another part of you, however, already feels tired from long work hours and poor sleep. It likes sitting on the couch because it likes the rest. The last thing it wants to do is go for a bike ride or a jog.

Psychologists call the state where part of you wants to do one thing and another part wants to do the opposite, cognitive dissonance. Usually, your Surface Brain has a list of rational, logical reasons for why it wants to make positive change, and the Deep Brain has its own list, usually less rational, for why it doesn't. Because the Deep Brain doesn't speak in words, it can sometimes be difficult to determine these hidden obstacles.

Sometimes we don't recognize these obstacles simply because we haven't taken the time to acknowledge them. In this case, simply ask yourself, "Why do I not want to (fill in the blank)?" Be completely honest with yourself.

At other times, it may not be so obvious. Look at your past behaviors for clues as to what your Deep Brain really wants and how it has opposed your efforts. Listen to your gut feelings.

Cognitive dissonance and its hidden obstacles is a common reason why we fail to achieve our goals or desired changes. Ignoring those hidden needs is not an effective strategy. Your Deep Brain is too strong for that. The most effective way to move forward is to provide for your hidden needs in healthier ways.

What needs are your current unhealthy, unwanted behaviors and habits meeting? What can you do to meet those needs in healthier ways?

Not all obstacles are hidden deep within your subconscious mind, and many of them can easily be predicted and dealt with before they happen. It's usually better to have a contingency plan in place before we become overwhelmed by a problem. In the heat of an adverse situation, much of your Surface Brain's rational capacity may be consumed, thus limiting your ability to think creatively, divergently and comprehensively.

Contingency planning is a large part of flying safely. As a private pilot, I fly single-engine airplanes. Over the years, I have had numerous small issues arise, like radio and alternator failures. When flying small, single-engine airplanes, it's not a question of *if* you are going to have a problem, it's a matter of *when*. Fortunately, I have never had any life-threatening issues arise. With that said, all pilots are taught to practice various predefined procedures to prevent and deal with potential problems. One way we plan for contingent problems is to select alternate airports during the flight planning process. I list the alternate airports in the order they occur along my flight path and all the needed radio frequencies for each so I have quick access to them. As I fly, I am also constantly thinking about where I could land if I couldn't make one of those alternate airports.

It's common to encounter problems during high-workload segments of flight, such as takeoff or landing. Many private pilots have forgotten to lower their landing gear simply because they became distracted or overwhelmed. I could choose to ignore this and hope for the best, or I could plan accordingly. I always use landing and takeoff checklists to help keep me from making such mistakes. Forming your own checklists is a good way to pre-plan for events that may overwhelm your ability to think clearly and comprehensively.

Mike Tyson said, "Everybody has a plan until they get punched in the mouth."[94] Life can sometimes be even more brutal. Even your best plans will need contingencies. Like flying, it's not a question of if things will go wrong. It's a question of when they will go wrong.

When you are in the midst of one of life's storms, it can be difficult to think clearly. Neurocognitive scientists recommend you develop a set of what they call "implementation intentions" or "when-then strategies." An implementation intention outlines what action you will take when an obstacle arises. Think of these as checklists for living.

Say you've started a diet and have been invited to a party where you know they will be serving all sorts of tasty, high-calorie finger foods. You know you will be a little hungry and thus vulnerable. A reasonable implementation intention would be to take a low-calorie food with you or eat something healthy before you go. This way you are not solely depending on your willpower to bail you out in the middle of a mounting temptation.

One of literature's most famous stories of implementation intentions is that of Odysseus and the famed island of the Sirens. Homer wrote that while Odysseus was sailing home after the Trojan War, he had to pass dangerously close to the island. He had been forewarned that the Sirens' songs were so enticing no man could resist, and sailors were lured to shipwreck on the rocky coast. Odysseus wanted to hear the famous Sirens, but was wisely afraid of their power. As his boat approached, he requested that his men tie him to the mast and ordered them not to release him no matter how much he pleaded. He then instructed them to fill their ears with beeswax so they could not hear the Sirens' call.

---

94 Mike Berardino, *Mike Tyson Explains One of His Most Famous Quotes* (South Florida Sun-Sentinel, November 8, 2012).

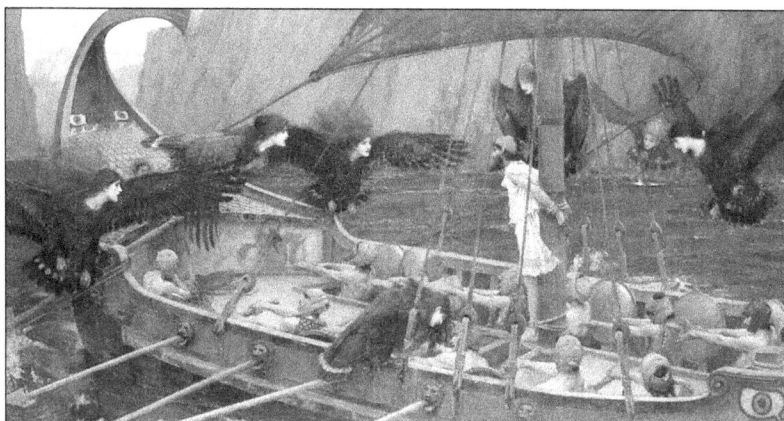

(FIGURE 7.7)[95]

Action Steps

Identify the benefits of your unwanted behaviors and plan to meet those needs in healthier ways. List this in your Life Plan.

What other potential problems do you foresee arising as you attempt to make healthier changes? What alluring Sirens may tempt you to stray from your healthy path? Develop your own problem-solving checklists. List those in your Life Plan.

You may consider problem-solving with a friend or your mastermind group. A broader perspective could help you develop more comprehensive strategies.

It is important to not only think about these contingency plans, but to write them down, especially for your most important changes and the ones that you believe will be the most difficult.

95 Waterhouse, John, "Ulysses and the Sirens", Oil on canvas, 1891, National Gallery of Victoria, Melbourne, Australia, https://artsandculture.google.com/asset/ulysses-and-the-sirens/qQH6ni1OHjyz9A?hl=en.

12. Prioritize

As much as you may want, you will not be able to change everything at once. Human nature propels us to overestimate what we can accomplish in a day, and underestimate what we can accomplish in a year. Overwhelm is the enemy. Neuroscientists call this the "Planning Fallacy." Err on the side of starting small. Err on the side of accomplishing your most important tasks first.

In 1991, Billy Crystal, Daniel Stern, Bruno Kirby, and Jack Palance starred in the western comedy *City Slickers*. When Mitch, played by Crystal, turns thirty-nine, his two best friends take him on vacation to drive cattle for a working dude ranch from New Mexico to Colorado. All three men are struggling with their own midlife crises and think the adventure will be a good break from their normal lives. To their surprise, this respite from reality is filled with a series of mounting challenges. As they ride their horses, Curly, the crusty yet wise old cowboy trail boss played by Palance, turns to Mitch. He asks him if he knows the secret of life. When Mitch replies in the negative, Curly holds up one finger. Mitch is confused. One finger? Curly clarifies: one thing. When Mitch asks what this secret one thing is, Curly simply replies, "That's what you got to figure out."[96]

Years later, one of my best friends gave me a book by Gary Keller called *The One Thing*. The premise of the book is based on Curly's advice. Prioritize your life and accomplish the most important thing first. Once you do that, move on to the next thing. That book and its simple concept was one of the niduses for my own adventure. For me, the one thing began as a simple task: wake up five minutes early and put my exercise clothes on. That habit slowly grew to exercising for an hour five days of the week. Emboldened by my success, I began waking up even earlier to read. Eventually, what began as a simple decision

---

96   Ron Underwood, *City Slickers* (Columbia Pictures, June 7, 1991).

to wake up five minutes early led to me writing this book, opening my own gym and leaving the comfort of my traditional medical practice to start a smaller, more relationship-centric clinic. It continues to guide my decisions and my adventure continues to evolve.

Review all your Life Domains and the visions you have created for each. Select one or two which, if realized, would change your life in the most positive ways. If working toward two feels too overwhelming, start with just the one thing, as Curly suggested. Dedicate yourself to making those things happen. Success breeds success. Once you make progress toward your dreams, your success will empower and motivate you to tackle your other life visions.

I have also discovered that success also breeds clarity. A few things I thought were important at the time I wrote my first Life Plan are not relevant now. As I accomplished my most important tasks, I learned, I grew, new opportunities opened, and my vision and priorities shifted.

Action Steps

What are the one or two most important visions you want to accomplish? Write them down.

What are the very first action steps you need to take to begin to accomplish these visions? Write them down.

I recommend making these first steps "stupid simple." Simplify them so they are almost impossible to fail. As an example, one of my initial visions was to improve my physical fitness. My first stupid simple action step was to get out of bed five minutes early and get dressed for a morning walk. That's it. I didn't get on the treadmill or walk outside. Getting dressed was 100 percent a success, and I was 100 percent certain that I could do that. After a week of getting out of bed, getting dressed and then crawling back into bed, I felt empowered. I knew I could add another small increment. I included walking on my treadmill for five minutes. I only added anything new to the routine once I had enjoyed the motivating success of moving my dreams forward.

If you haven't already done so, rewrite your initial action steps so that they are stupid simple.

13. Schedule your first steps

Structure your time around your most important values. Wrap your personal visions and values with the activities of your daily life.

The most common time people set goals is on New Year's Eve. With the excitement of the parties and parades, the New Year always seems to start off with great potential. We map out how we're going to lose weight, get in shape, make more money, and stay in touch with family and friends. At the beginning of each year, our gym fills with new faces, but by April most of them are gone. These people had grand visions for their year, but along the way they became discouraged by the small progress relative to the size of their big vision.

Not only can you simplify the vision to small actions steps, you can also redefine the time frame on which you focus. Restructure your vision from, "What can I accomplish by the end of my life?" or even, "What can I accomplish in the next year?" to, "What can I accomplish in twelve weeks?"

Your lifetime is hopefully a long one, and while that grand vision may feel exciting it could also be a little overwhelming. I like to think in terms of what I can accomplish in the next twelve weeks. Twelve-week blocks are much more manageable. Once you complete your first twelve-week block, you tackle the next one.

Start by scheduling your first week. It is important to write your first simple action step on your calendar to clear space in your busy life so you have adequate time to accomplish the task. If you don't make time for it, your daily routine will choke out your dreams. Scheduling forces you to at least acknowledge that your time is limited.

Action Steps

Now you have decided which one or two visions are most important, define what you need to accomplish in the next twelve weeks to help move you toward those visions.

Schedule the first incredibly-simple-almost-impossible-to-fail first step on your calendar.

14. Get to work!

"A journey of 1,000 miles begins with a single step."[97]

Remember the tachometer in my Life Machine drawing. The "M" in "RPM" stands for movement. A goal without movement, without action, is just a fantasy.

What fears keep you standing on the sideline saying you'll achieve your dreams someday?

Life is like a diving platform; most people spend all their time climbing up and down the ladder. It makes them feel busy, but they don't accomplish anything. They never jump. Perpetually planning and dreaming makes us feel like we are accomplishing something, but the only people who accomplish anything are those who dive off into the abyss of the unknown. Standing on the edge of the platform can feel frightening. Nobody knows how people will react to their work. Your responsibility is to dive into the sea, to do the work, to face the fear, and jump anyway.

Action Step

Stop planning and start the actual work of changing your life. Unless you do something with your plan, all your work to date is pointless.

----

97 Lao Tzu (traditionally accredited), Dao de Jing, 4th century B.C.

15. Monitor and Adjust

Read your Life Plan, or at least the portions that you are actively working toward, daily for the next twelve weeks. Act and speak as if the story you are creating is already true. Reading your Life Plan daily helps you keep what you have deemed most important in the forefront of your mind. Acting and speaking as if your vision is already reality boosts your confidence and the belief that your vision will come true.

At the end of each week, and the end of each twelve-week block, set aside time to review your progress. What were your successes and struggles? What activities should you continue? What activities do you need to change? What are you feeling?

I like to do this on Sunday night. I review the week then I plan for the week to come, always making sure I schedule the most important activities first. Similar to Benjamin Franklin, I keep a diary with my thoughts and plans. I also adapted his chart of virtues to a large wall calendar which hangs in my home office. Each day that I accomplish my most important tasks, I mark a big red "X" on the calendar. As I link together a series of Xs, they form a chain. My goal is consistency— don't break the chain. My goal has been to write 500-1,000 words of this book a day. Writing a 90,000-word book can feel daunting, but writing 500 words a day is manageable. Seeing my chain grow keeps me motivated and accountable.

Another important concept to keep in mind is that your Life Plan should remain flexible. None of us has the power to see into the future. Your Life Plan will provide you with direction, but as you proceed you will learn more about yourself, and if you pay attention you will discover opportunities you would not have predicted. As you learn, update your visions and change direction accordingly. When I wrote my first Life Plan several years ago, one of my goals was to maintain 6-8 percent body fat. I dropped down to about 9 percent but after a few months I decided that goal really wasn't important. I feel better around 15 percent body fat, a much more reasonable goal for me.

When I was young and learning to swim, my father would encourage me to jump into the pool and swim to him. Typically, he would tread water just three or four feet from the edge which didn't seem too hard to reach, but as soon as I jumped in he began swimming backward. My target was moving. I couldn't control that. All I could do was keep swimming. Before I knew it, I'd swam the length of the entire pool, much further than I thought I could have ever done at the beginning.

Sometimes the vision continuously expands so that it remains just out of your grasp. Sometimes life changes it for you, and sometimes you will do everything as well as you possibly can and still fall short. Remember the vision is only a beacon. It is something you aim toward, but it is not the final destination. The path of progress—the way—is the destination. The work you do as you travel toward the destination—the vision—is all you can ultimately control.

Living a beautiful life is about continuously grasping a little farther than you can reach, always hoping and striving for a better, more exciting tomorrow while enjoying the fullness and beauty of the present moment. Reviewing your progress and adjusting your visions will help keep you motivated and ensure you continue to head in the right direction.

The Self-Care Journal

My Self-Care Journal is a practical tool I use to help me create, monitor and adjust my Life Plan. As you can see below, I divide my entries into three timeframes: the morning entries, the evening entries and the end of the week/beginning of a new week entries. Don't feel you need to strictly follow the time schedule that I use or that you must include all portions for your Self-Care Journal to work. I fluctuate, placing more emphasis on some portions at times, skipping some entirely at others, while always trying to focus on those that seem most pertinent at the time.

Self-Care Journal Outline

I. Morning

1. **Freewrite:** For several minutes, write down all your spontaneous thoughts. Don't edit, just write. I find this a great way to loosen my creativity and develop new insights.

2. **Gratitude writing:** Write about three things for which you are thankful. Force yourself to identify and write about three new things each day.

3. **Review your To-Dos for the day:** Have you prioritized the things you need to accomplish? Most of us place more on our To-Do list than we can possibly achieve. Remember The One Thing. Have you defined the next most important specific action step you need to accomplish to move toward your grand vision? Have you set aside a specific time on your calendar to achieve it?

4. **Mood journal:** Identify difficult emotions and negative thoughts (this may need to be an ongoing process throughout the day.) Process and dispute them with the tools you learned from Chapters Three and Four. Writing is a powerful tool that can help you process them, especially when you are first learning the tools.

5. **Life Plan Review:** Read a segment of your Life Plan every morning. The old adage "out of sight out of mind" applies here. You want to keep your vision alive in your mind. This helps you focus on what is important.

II. Evening

1. **Review your day:** What did you **D**iscover, **A**chieve, are you **T**hankful for or **E**xcited about? (Remember the acronym **DATE**.) Write a few sentences about these in your journal.

2. **Plan for the next day:** Set priorities. Schedule specific action steps from your To-Do list. Place them on your calendar.

3. **Monitor Specific Behaviors:** Have you identified markers to track your progress? How did you do today? This week? Record them now: diet log, weight chart, number of pages read, miles walked or hours slept.

4. **Mood journal:** Review what you wrote earlier in the day and add any negative thoughts and emotions you want to explore and work through.

III. End of the week/Start of the new week

1. **Review the Week:** List all your major highlights and struggles. What can you celebrate? What can you learn?

2. **Set intentions for the next week:** Review what you want to accomplish this upcoming week. Prioritize your list.

3. **Schedule your specific action steps:** Make room on your calendar for your most important activities.

My Lack of Planning

As I look back at the tragedy of Amelia Earhart, it's easy to criticize her for planning poorly. The truth is, I am guilty of similar mistakes. I've just been lucky enough that my poor planning hasn't cost me my life. In 2004, my family and I went on vacation to Colorado. Our first stop was Durango. At the time, I was obsessed with mountain biking.

I usually took my bike everywhere, but for some reason I left it at home on this trip.

Durango is one of the birthplaces of mountain biking and the home of one of the sport's early legends, Ned Overend. To say that I was excited is a complete understatement. The very first thing I did was to leave my family, on our family vacation, and run to a local bike store to rent a mountain bike. That was my first mistake.

The shop owner gave me a map of an epic local ride, and I set off on my adventure. This was in the early days of cellphones, so I reasoned that there would be no coverage in this remote area and left our only phone for my wife. My second mistake.

I was confident in my abilities. On any given day, if you asked me to ride 100-150 miles, I could do it. I was in the best shape of my entire life. I knew riding solo was a little risky, but ego beat reason. My third mistake.

I also did not account for the altitude. I lived and trained in Tyler, Texas, which has an elevation of 540 feet. Durango's elevation is 6,500 feet and the mountains I was cycling toward were even higher. This was my first day at altitude and after just a few minutes, I knew I was in trouble. Typically after about thirty minutes of riding, my body settles into a comfortable pace, but I was struggling. My heart was racing, and I remember feeling my carotid arteries pounding like they were about to explode. My breathing was labored, and my balance seemed off. None of this deterred me, however. I assumed I would just pedal through it. My fourth mistake.

I wasn't only struggling with the altitude; I was struggling with my rental bike and pedals. The bike was a little small and handled differently from my usual one. The mechanism for releasing my feet from the pedals was also different enough that I couldn't release my feet automatically. I had to consciously think about it, which delayed my release. None of these issues were much of a problem by themselves, but compounded by the altitude and overconfidence, they set the stage for my story.

After a couple hours of riding, I fatigued prematurely. My riding became sloppy and less precise. Recovering from a steep climb, I barreled down the opposite side. As I rounded a sandy curve at the bottom, my back tire started sliding. Even some sixteen years later, I can see all of this in slow motion. "No problem," I thought. A little adjustment and the bike will be back on track—except it didn't respond. The bike flew one direction and I the other with my right foot still bound to the pedal. In midair, I felt and heard my leg snap. I knew it was broken before I even hit the ground.

"What just happened?" I thought. I was stunned. After a few minutes of lying on the ground, the reality of my situation registered. I was in trouble. Out here, I was part of the food chain and I had quickly slipped to the bottom. Miles from civilization, with no way to call and no fellow rider to help me, I did what any reasonable person would do. I screamed. Surprise, surprise—nobody heard me. Eventually, I stood to see if I could locate any riders who could come to my aid. The entire valley below was visible. Several miles in the distance, the dust plumes of two riders rose from the valley floor. Nobody was going to hear me. I was on my own.

Pedaling was not possible. Using the bike as a crutch, I hopped up the next hill. Exhausted and frustrated, a combination of bravery and fear of impending nightfall compelled me to try to coast down the hill. Mounting my bike with my right leg held out to the side, my speed gradually increased. "This is going to work," I thought. "I'm going to make it." Then out of nowhere my leg, broken and extended to the side, collided with a tree. I think I blacked out for a moment. Once again, I found myself face down in the dirt, but fear of being stuck in the wilderness at night motivated me to jump back on the bike again. "Jump" may be a strong term. "Cautiously climbed" might be a better description. For hours, I repeated the process, hopping up one hill and coasting down the next. Two more times, angry trees grabbed my leg and threw me back to the ground.

I was well past my agreed-upon return time. My wife and children, fearful that something serious had happened, started up the trail to find me. Along the way, I passed them as I coasted down a hill. I didn't stop but yelled, "I broke my leg and need to go to the hospital." I think I was more afraid of my wife's wrath, so not stopping seemed like another good idea at the time. Chalk that up to another poor decision.

Overconfidence in my abilities, and a history of successes with previous near misses, lulled me into complacency. I had no way to communicate and nobody to help me. I had no contingency plan for emergencies. See the overlap with Earhart? I was fortunate. Unlike Earhart my crash wasn't fatal, but it could have been much worse than it was. Luck was on my side that day.

To help remind me of the crash, like I will ever forget, my wife had a caricature made of me in my "proud" moment (Figure 7.8.) She thought I needed a memento to remind me of my less-than-smart series of decisions.

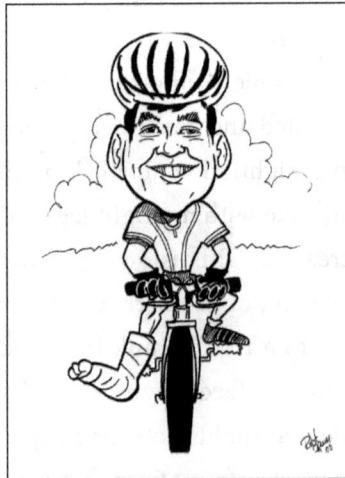

(FIGURE 7.8)

I learn the most when I fall and find myself face down in the dirt—Adversity. Unfortunately, it has taken several crashes to grab my attention.

What "crashes" have you experienced that could have been prevented if you had planned a little better? What lessons did you learn from those experiences? How can you use them to positively plan for your future? On what exciting adventures have you always wanted to embark, but were too afraid that you may crash? Sit down today and begin to write your Life Plan.

Summary

- Self-control is a combination of thought control, emotional control, impulse control, and performance control. All are dependent on a Common Mental Energy Resource (CMER.)

- Living a beautiful life requires you to use your CMER judiciously and frequently replenish it.

- Writing a Life Plan will help you clarify, prioritize and allocate your limited CMERs.

- Like pilots who develop a thorough flight plan and authors who outline their story, developing a Life Plan will help ensure you reach your desired destination.

- **Summary for writing your Life Plan:**

  1. Time to Think: Schedule time alone to think and write your plan.

  2. Aged Portrait: Download an app and create an aged picture of yourself.

  3. A Better Version of You: Look into the eyes of your aged self and listen to the advice they would give you. Imagine this version of yourself is surrounded by the people you care

about most—what are the life stories you want them to reminisce about? What does a well-lived life look like from your aged self's perspective? Write a few paragraphs that summarize these stories.

4. Life Domains: Define your ten most important Life Domains.

5. Destination: Create an exciting vision for each of your Life Domains.

6. Note the Gap: On scale from -10 to +10, subjectively rank how well you are achieving your vision for each domain. Mark this on your Dream Assessment Tool. This notes your current reality. Be honest with yourself and note the difference between where you are and where you want to go.

7. Purpose: As you write the narrative for each of your Life Domains, note how each of them helps you accomplish your sacred task, your purpose, your meaningful work. What skills and competencies must you develop for each? What activities will help you produce not just simple results but exponential results? Take a few minutes and write about these.

8. Allies: What people do you need to include in your journey? Make a list of them and intentionally reach out. Whose content do you need to consume more of? Make a list of the books, articles and videos you think will help you develop into the person you want to become. Set aside deliberate time to consume this content. Summarize their recommendations and write down a few of their most inspirational quotations.

9. SMARTER Steps: Create a series of smaller, SMARTER steps that will help you progress toward your grander vision for each domain.

10. Obstacles: What internal and external obstacles may arise to thwart your progress? What benefits are your current un-

wanted behaviors providing for you? How can you meet your needs in healthier ways? What external factors are most likely to hinder your progress? Write out your contingency plans.

11. Prioritize: Select the one or two most important tasks that if accomplished would change your life in the most positive ways.

12. Time to Schedule: Simplify your one or two most important visions into what you think you can accomplish in the next twelve weeks.

13. Get to Work: Time to stop all the planning and jump into completing the tasks.

14. Monitor and Adjust: How will you know when you have accomplished your task? Is it specific? Is it measurable? If not, go back to SMARTER steps and refine them so you have something concrete you can monitor. At the same time, remain flexible and adjust your efforts as your vision morphs and expands.

• Consider starting a Self-Care Journal. I found this to be a practical tool that helps me create, monitor and adjust my Life Plan.

We have come a long way since the beginning of the book. For a moment, let's return to the introduction where I discussed the concept of Empowered Self-Care. You can now see how conserving CMER is a common thread that links all of these strategies (Figure 7.9.)

Adversity: Challenges are common to us all, but whether we suffer because of them is in large part due to how we manage our automatic, Deep Brain reactions.

Awareness: Living in a healthy, balanced emotional state consumes less CMER than constantly suppressing and controlling difficult emotions.

Attenuation: Quickly disputing automatic negative thoughts consumes less CMER than continuously fighting the undertows of recirculating negative thoughts.

Assets: Performing tasks at which you are naturally gifted consumes less CMER than tasks at which you are not.

Allies: Living in environments and around people who positively support you consumes less CMER than living in environments and around people who thwart your efforts to grow and achieve.

Aim: Following a clear and concise plan conserves CMER, saving your limited mental resources for those difficult moments when you may need all the mental capacity you find.

In the final chapter, **Action,** we will discuss how to tie all these concepts into a single unified effort. It is all about Getting to Work, deliberately choosing and carrying out the behaviors and activities that enrich, restore and replenish your CMER. Efficiently using your limited CMER is a common thread that links all of our strategies for living well.

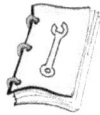

Empowered Self-Care

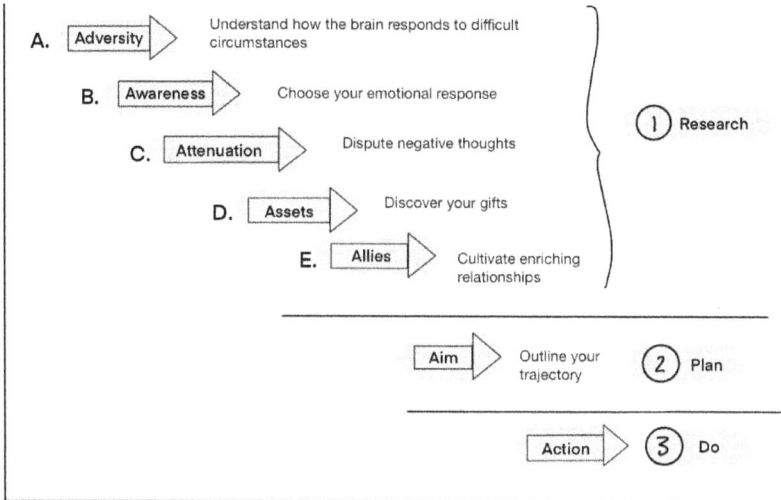

A. Adversity — Understand how the brain responds to difficult circumstances

B. Awareness — Choose your emotional response

C. Attenuation — Dispute negative thoughts

D. Assets — Discover your gifts

E. Allies — Cultivate enriching relationships

① Research

Aim — Outline your trajectory

② Plan

Action

③ Do

(FIGURE 7.9)

CHAPTER 8

Action — Act With Persistence and Intent

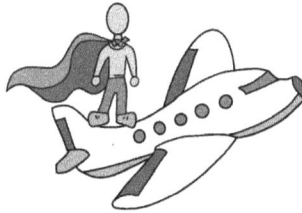

ARRIVAL GATE 1A: Adversity

DEPARTURE GATE 6A: Awareness, Attenuation, Assets, Allies, Aim, Action

Boarding Pass	Empowered Self-Care	Boarding Pass
Username: _____ **First Class**		← ☑ Departures
Destination: Beautiful Life Current Location: Reality		✈ **6A**
Arrival: **Gate 1A** (Adversity)		Gate
Departure: **Gate 6A** (Awareness, Attenuation, Assets, Allies, Aim, Action)		

Most people think: they can think themselves to health and happiness.

The truth is: action is the root of opportunity and healing. Opportunities are revealed as a function of steps taken, not intentions deliberated.

"I find the great thing in this world is not so much where we stand, as in what direction we are moving. To reach the port of heaven, we must sail sometimes with the wind and sometimes against it—but we must sail, and not drift, nor lie at anchor."[98]

"You cannot discover new oceans until you have the courage to lose sight of the shore."[99]

"If opportunity doesn't knock, build a door."[100]

Terry walks into my office slightly hunched over, emotionless and reluctant to make eye contact. He appears defeated and depressed. For the last few years his family and I have noticed a slow decline in his mood. A once engaging and creative middle school music teacher, Terry has progressively become cynical, angry and morose. Like most young people, he began his career with optimism, feeling like he could positively change the education system and, more importantly, help shape the lives of young people. Over time, the bureaucracy of the education system wore him down, now Terry says he simply goes through the motions, doing what he has to do to keep his job and provide for his family.

His wife says Terry can't stop complaining about work. He says the school system negatively impacts his life and mishandles childrens' potential. In the past, she enjoyed listening to him play his

98 Oliver Wendell Holems, Sr., *The Autocrat of the Breakfast-Table*, (iOnlineShopping.com. February 20. 2019).

99 Anonymous.

100 Milton Berle Quotes, BrainyQuote.com, BrainyMedia Inc, 2022, https://www.brainyquote.com/quotes/milton_berle_105306.

piano and write music in his home studio. That is one of the many things that originally attracted her to him, but over the last few years he has stopped playing. She says he always seems bitter and angry, frequently taking his frustrations out on her and the children. She confides in me that while she still loves Terry, she is not sure how much more she can take.

Terry knows his attitude has become toxic and difficult to live with, but says, "I can't seem to pull myself out of it." He feels more and more distant from his wife and children, yet finds himself saying and doing things that only worsen the problem. "Life seems pointless," he says, "I've given up on my music making a difference and I've lost my creative voice, so I just stopped playing. These days when I come home I surf the internet and sip scotch until I fall asleep in my recliner. I get up in the morning, go to work and repeat it all again. Truthfully, I'm just waiting. I'm just biding time. I don't want to hurt myself, but it'd be okay if I didn't wake up."

Once an active member in his church, Terry no longer finds comfort in the services or the companionship and communal experience of worship. He has withdrawn from friends and they from him, in part because his attitude is so toxic that few people want to spend time with him. He is depressed and sees no positive path forward.

Introduction of Empowered Self-Care

Over the years, Terry has tried several different antidepressant medications. While each was mildly effective, none of them cured his depression and agitation. Terry has been skeptical about psychology and repeatedly has declined my recommendations for him to see a counselor, which has hindered his progress even more.

Hoping to make inroads, I take a different approach. We discuss how recent neuroscience discoveries suggest that the adult brain is more malleable than we once believed. As we have now learned, changing the way we think physically alters the brain's electrical circuits. Chronic reactive ways of thinking and responding can be "rewired" with the right tools, helping the brain process and respond to adversities in healthier ways. This concept of "rewiring the brain" seems to intrigue Terry, and I use this small window as an opportunity to introduce the concepts of Empowered Self-Care. I offer its components as a list of tools from which he can choose, and encourage him to select the one that resonates most.

Adversity: Discover how the human brain responds to difficult circumstances.

Awareness: Learn how to recognize, embrace and choose your emotional responses.

Attenuation: Learn to recognize and dispute automatic negative thoughts.

Assets: Discover your natural strengths and gifts.

Allies: Cultivate enriching relationships and environments.

Aim: Compose a flexible map to guide you and keep you on task.

Action: Engage in activities to make progress toward your goals and positively change the way you think and feel.

I explain that all six categories are helpful and there is no one right place or way to start the journey.

After deliberating for a few minutes, Terry says the first few feel too "touchy-feely," besides he isn't so sure he is ready for all of that. Aiming seems reasonable, like something concrete he can do right now. To begin the process I ask him to list his most important 8-10 Life Domains and review how to write a Life Plan as discussed in Chapter 7. For his "homework," I ask him to spend the next couple of weeks composing a Life Plan based on these domains.

When Terry returns about three weeks later he has completed his Life Plan and identified the two most important things he wants to begin working on. For him, the most important task to begin is to become a better husband and father. He knows his wife is thinking about leaving him and is afraid that if things don't turn around quickly, he is going to lose her. He isn't sure if he will be able to survive that loss.

We discuss a few principles of building and maintaining healthy relationships and emphasize that his work is to focus on changing himself, not trying to change his wife. I also remind him that as he becomes the version of himself that she needs him to be, he not only helps her, but heals himself as well. I like to say, "As **USAVE** yourself, **USAVE** your partner."

USAVE is an acronym I use to help me remember and focus my attention on several tools to build and maintain healthy relationships.

U: Understand. Seek first to understand your partner's

- Hopes and dreams
- Strengths and values
- Enduring vulnerabilities
- Wants and needs

S: Stay connected. We depart our relationships in malicious and mindless ways. Malicious exits are easy to see, but mindless exits are more insidious and difficult to recognize. They may even be disguised as good activities like working, spending time with the children or volunteering. Be mindful of how you and your partner exit the relationship in both ways and make deliberate attempts to close them. Staying connected also reminds us that in times of conflict, forging new, healthier versions of the relationship is an important step of forgiving.

A: Affirm. We must deliberately search for and affirm our partner's positive traits both to them (outwardly) and to ourselves (inwardly.) As part of my morning meditation, I list and remind myself of the positive traits of the people with whom I may be in conflict.

Most people who are harshly critical of others are also harshly critical of themselves. If we feel inadequate about ourselves then we are in constant search for what is not there in ourselves as well as what is absent in others. As part of the affirmation process, therefore, it is also helpful to deliberately search for and self-affirm your positive traits as well as the positive traits of others.

V: Validate. Validation is a practical way of showing compassion and understanding, especially during conflict.

- Use the way you listen to acknowledge that what your partner says is important.

- Ask open-ended questions and ask your partner to elaborate as well as give examples in an attempt to understand.

- Reflect back to your partner what they say. You can do this by repeating exactly what they say or paraphrasing so they can hear their thoughts through your voice.

- Once they finish sharing, ask if they have anything else they want to say, and if not offer a brief summary.

- Attempt to view the issue from their perspective. Share that even though you may disagree, you can see how their thoughts make sense, or that their thoughts seem logical when you look at it from their point of view.

- Finally, it is important to validate their feelings. If your partner is telling you something they're upset about, they're most often not seeking advice to solve the problem. They simply want to feel understood. Don't try to fix their problem, but pay attention to the emotion they are expressing. Tell them something like, "I can understand how that would make you feel sad/angry/jealous/confused/frustrated," or, "I can see how that hurt you."

Identify the emotion they are experiencing and let them clearly know that you recognize it.

E: Engage. Relationships become enriching when we do things that cause our partner to view us as a source of fun, safety and support.

- **Caring Behaviors:** Ask your partner to list the things they would like you to do for them:

  - Things you are doing now that they would like you to continue doing and do more often.

  - Things you have done in the past they would like you to restart.

  - Things you have never done that they want you to start doing

- **Surprise List:** Pay attention to things or activities that your partner wants, but never specifically asks for, and surprise them with them.

- **SMART Requests:** During times of conflict it is important to state what you need in clear, concise and reasonable ways. Make a list of up to three things that you want your partner to do differently. Ask them to rank your requests from easiest to hardest and allow them to choose which request they are willing to do.

- **Fun Activities:** Spend time engaging in activities you mutually enjoy. Most people will find that unless they deliberately make a list of activities and intentionally set time aside for them, the busyness of life will passively fill their time.

Implementation

With "Relationships" identified as his most important Life Domain, Terry narrows it further to salvaging his marriage and, after our conversation, implements what he jokingly refers to as, "Project USAVE." He identifies work, scotch and TV as the primary ways he passively exits his marriage, and begins to make a conscious effort to reverse that. He also recognizes that he isn't a good listener and that by always trying to fix his wife's problems he is negating her thoughts and feelings. Terry also introduces a few activities, like re-establishing a weekly date night and surprising his wife with small gifts.

These initial efforts produce positive results and his wife begins to notice, which encourages Terry to commit even more to the process. Terry and I continue to meet every 2-4 weeks over the next year and work through the other components in Empowered Self-Care. He becomes more **aware** of his emotional complexity, as well as the complexity of his wife and others. He begins to identify his own internal voices of distorted thinking and to **attenuate** them to healthier levels. Instead of dwelling on his inadequacies, he acknowledges and focuses on what is right and beautiful about himself, his **assets.** He decides to unapologetically live into his natural gifts and starts writing and playing music again.

As Terry learns more, he decides to start a mens' group where he can surround himself with **allies** who will support each other as they attempt to grow. As Terry intentionally **aims** his life in a healthier direction, he modifies his Life Plan to reflect newly discovered opportunities and ways to progressively grow.

Crisis

Things are improving and Terry makes consistent strides forward for several months, but then he hits a hard wall. As with most progress, growth is uneven. Terry has done well, but recently slumped into some of his old habits and distorted ways of thinking. His wife, who had been so encouraged initially, now feels betrayed, saying that Terry is now even more aggressive, agitated and angry than he has ever been. Completely discouraged, she rents an apartment and moves out with the children.

While Terry has made progress, his self-care work brought diffi-cult emotions and thoughts he'd worked hard to suppress for decades to the surface. His new "head knowledge," as he likes to say, has begun to shed light on the root of his anger, shame and blame, but they are still smoldering beneath the surface. He is still learning how to use his self-care tools to combat them, but despite his efforts he begins to feel overwhelmed. Scotch, work and numbing return like faithful old friends.

As Terry shares what is happening, he offers that his childhood was, "complicated, but not unusual." His parents were, "fine, upstand-ing, church-going people." On the outside they seemed to have everything together, but at home their relationship was toxic, and it spilled over into the way they treated their children. Terry says his mother probably lived with bipolar disorder. He never knew which version would greet him from one moment to the next. Sometimes she would be overly affectionate and clingy; the next moment she would yell and scream in fits of rage. He still remembers the first time he felt "unadulterated hate" as he looked into her eyes. He is quick to add that she never physically abused him, but he never felt safe with her. "As soon as I allowed myself to get close, she would attack and pull the rug out from under me." According to Terry, his mother had been physically, emotionally and sexually abused by her own father and had never learned how to cope with it. This left her particularly distrustful and resentful toward men in general. She was also dis-trustful of modern-day psychology, preferring to explain her pain and responses in simplistic black-and-white terms. "You were either good or bad, with her or against her, agreed with her or were wrong. There was no middle ground."

Terry says his father was stuck in an old paternalistic view of marriage, one where he saw himself as the head of the household and everyone else was to subjugate themselves to him. He, like Terry's mother, viewed the world from a dogmatic, dichotomous, simplest perspective that left little room for disagreement. He prided himself in his intellectual ability to debate, viewing relationships as something to conquer. You either won and survived or you lost and died. There was only room in a relationship for one person to be right and to dominate.

As you could expect, Terry's mother, who had been abused by her father, was in no way interested in being mistreated by another man and so their marriage was filled with constant fighting and turmoil. Terry's father had no good role models for healthy relationships either, so the sins of one generation were passed onto the next.

Terry's father also thought modern psychology was stuck in its Freudian theories. His parents had sought the counsel of a well-intentioned pastor who ultimately had no good solutions and told them they both simply had "strong personalities." With no tools to help them repair their marriage, they gave up on the relationship. While they prided themselves for not divorcing, they both exited the relationship emotionally long ago, thereby creating a silent divorce.

Terry's father found sanctuary in his work, spending almost twenty-four hours a day away from the family except on weekends. As the oldest male figure in the house, Terry was left to fend for himself against his mother who seemed to both love and despise the two most prominent male figures in her life. As a child, Terry didn't know how to cope, so he emotionally distanced himself from them both, and found anger and achievement as ways to protect himself and find affection.

Isolating vulnerable feelings, anger and achievement guided Terry safely through his childhood but as a thirty-five-year-old father, husband and teacher, his old coping skills are now causing more harm than good. He's not only losing the relationships he cherishes most, but losing his ability to think critically, expansively and creatively. His depression and pessimism are blinding him to creative opportunities and solutions, and his sense of worthlessness, victimhood, blame, and shame deepens.

Just like his father, Terry initially used work as a refuge from his deteriorating marriage, but stressors began to mount there as well. With no healthy way to cope, work became yet another trigger that propelled him into an emotional abyss.

Forgiving

Terry acknowledges that the resentment he still holds for his parents taints his overall attitude. He is profoundly disappointed and disillusioned with them and the beliefs that fostered such caustic ways of treating others, and yet he finds himself repeating many of the same behaviors. Terry, more now than ever before, feels the weight of a pain that is as much about what happened as it is grief for the loss of what could have been.

When Terry tries to share his feelings and new self-care tools with his parents, they aren't interested in listening. His mother becomes defensive, and tells him that she doesn't have any problems and is not interested in changing. She says that he is arrogant and unappreciative of all their sacrifices.

Terry's father continues his passive approach of ignoring the problem. Instead of rebuilding a healthier relationship, he blames Terry for having an "unforgiving spirit." It seems to Terry that they have no safe and healthy way to process the truth and its associated discomfort, so it is easier for them to simply ignore it.

Terry wants to forgive and move past the pain, but the simple advice he had been taught and is still being given by friends and other family members isn't working. "Forgive and forget," "You have to move on," "You just need to pray about it more," all seem incomplete. While Terry knows they all mean well, their advice seems to dishonor his struggle and the genuine work he is attempting to do. Terry is confused. It doesn't make sense. How do you simply forget what happened? How do you move forward when the people who hurt you show no remorse and continue to hurt you? Burying his resentment and pain had only created more resentment and pain which had now come to a tipping point. Terry is searching for better answers.

I feel Terry's frustration and pain. Studies show that even if we simply attempt to ignore or "forget" the explicit memory of traumatic events, the emotional pain still lives deep in our subconscious neural systems, our Deep Brain, where it continues to actively shape our responses, beliefs and thoughts. These deep implicit memories are still alive, and burying living things is never a good idea.

When you ignore your pain without appropriately addressing it, it festers and grows. Because burying living things is by definition pathologic, the things we use to bury our pain also take on pathologic roles: work, scotch, sex, drugs, perfectionism, achievement, money, fame, power. Not dealing with one problem compounds the original issue by creating additional negative downstream consequences.

So how can you forgive and move past the pain of previous transgressions? How do you replace implicit memories that are encoded deep within your nervous system?

Tutu's Story

As I thought about Terry's dilemma and the similar ones we all face at points, I was reminded of Archbishop Desmond Tutu's story. Tutu became the de facto face of the struggle against apartheid in South

Africa as other political leaders like Nelson Mandela were imprisoned or killed. Tutu, a pastor in the Anglican church, saw himself as a simple preacher trying to lead his church through difficult times, yet found himself becoming the interim leader of the Black liberation struggle during the most tumultuous years of apartheid. He won the Nobel Peace Prize for this leadership.

Tutu was committed to finding a non-violent solution to end apartheid, and often found himself in precarious positions as he denounced the atrocities committed by state-controlled security forces while trying to calm angry mobs from issuing violent retribution. These mobs especially loathed informants that grew among their own ranks whom they called "impimpis." A particularly cruel form of execution called necklacing was exacted for these impipis. A car tire was placed around the victim's neck, filled with gasoline and then set on fire. On at least two occasions, Tutu thrust his own body between the victim and the frenzied mob to stop the executions.

Apartheid began to dismantle on February 2, 1990 when President Frederik Willem de Klerk unbanned all Black political movements and announced the release of Nelson Mandela and all other political leaders. Tutu says, however, he faced his most challenging task in the next phase. In December of 1995, he was appointed chairman of the South African Truth and Reconciliation Commission which was established to help heal the country.

Tutu believed that reconciliation and healing could only begin with the process of forgiveness. This did not mean trying to hide the ugly sins committed. In *The Book of Forgiveness* Tutu and his daughter Mpho shared several of the tragic stories presented to the commission that typified the atrocities committed under apartheid and by angry vigilante mobs looking for revenge. It opens with the story of a woman and her young daughter whose husband/father Sicelo disappeared. When his body was found, he had been stabbed forty-three times, had acid poured on his face, and his right hand severed.

Babalwa, who had been eight when her father was murdered, was now nineteen. Standing in front of the commission, she described the grief, police harassment and hardship that followed after her father's murder. Then she said, "I would love to know who killed my father. So would my brother. We want to forgive them. We want to forgive, but we don't know who to forgive."[101]

I'm not sure I would be able to forgive like this, and wonder what type of process Tutu espoused that could facilitate such forgiveness. How does someone begin to forgive the brutal murderers of their husband, father or child? Where do you even begin? This is the type of forgiveness I wanted to learn. It sounded much more healing than the simple advice I and others like Terry had been taught.

An Extended Path of Forgiveness

As Tutu explained his understanding of forgiveness, he reminded us that, "There is nothing that cannot be forgiven, and there is no one undeserving of forgiveness."[102] People often skip over their own and others' suffering and encourage others to shortcut the process of forgiveness. They go straight to words of forgiveness out of a perfunctory obligation for doing "the right thing." Spoken words of forgiveness that have not taken root in the heart, however, are what Tutu calls a "Veneer of Peace." That rang true to me, and seemed to be what Terry was also struggling with. People often push us or rush us through the stages of forgiveness and apply this veneer either because they don't understand the process themselves or have their own agendas. Nobody has the right to do that.

Tutu suggested that forgiveness is a fourfold path:

- Telling the story

---

101 Desmond Tutu and Mpho Tutu, *The Book of Forgiving* (HarperOne, March 18, 2014).
102 Desmond Tutu and Mpho Tutu, *The Book of Forgiving* (HarperOne, March 18, 2014).

- Naming the hurt
- Granting forgiveness
- Renewing or releasing the relationship

I compared Tutu's path of forgiveness to what I found in recent scientific studies, other faith based teachings, history, and literary works and settled on a similar common path to forgiveness. It begins by clearly stating what forgiveness is not.

Forgiveness is not:

- Pardoning the offender
- Relaxing the demands for justice
- Forgetting the wrong
- Condoning or excusing the offense
- Justifying
- Assuming that time will heal
- Ignoring the natural consequences of the offense

The mnemonic **A**nyone **C**an **F**orgive describes the path.

A: Acknowledge and Accept the facts and feelings. The truth must be brought to light. Shame and blame hide and grow in the shadows. When a perpetrator tells someone, "Never speak about this," they are desperately trying to hide their guilt. We must speak the truth, especially when it is uncomfortable.

C: Compose a coherent and compassionate explanation of your perpetrator's acts and your response.

F: Forge a healthier, more respectful version of the relationship. This may mean that you re-establish the relationship as one that recognizes healthier boundaries, but in the event the perpetrator is not willing or able to recognize these boundaries, you may choose to release the relationship.

1. Acknowledge and Accept

You may not be able to face your perpetrator for many reasons. They may be dead or in prison. They may not be interested in talking to you, or you may not feel physically or emotionally safe talking to them. Even if you cannot share the facts and feelings of your situation with the perpetrator directly, acknowledging them to yourself will help you heal. It can also be helpful to share your story with a compassionate friend. Choose somebody who will truly listen and not try to fix your situation or give you advice. If you don't have anybody like that, write your story as a letter. You don't need to send it to anybody, but this will help you process the pain.

Remember Kristin Neff's work with compassion we discussed in Chapter 3. Our natural instinct is to resist difficult circumstances and emotions. We don't like the way they make us feel, so we ignore them or bury them. Healing begins by becoming curious and exploring your adverse situation, starting with the facts and feelings. As we explore, we transition through tolerating, allowing and eventually befriending the adversity. As we befriend, we accept and let go of the need for the past and the perpetrator to be different from who they were and continue to be. You don't condone their behavior by accepting it, but this unshackles you from any need for the perpetrator to take action. This type of forgiveness is your path to choose and is not dependent on anybody else's action.

One note on acknowledging and accepting: I am not saying your perpetrator should not be punished for their actions, and I am not saying you should not try to stop them from acting in toxic ways. When somebody hurts us or others, they also hurt themselves. Stopping them may, therefore, be the most compassionate thing to do not only for you and others, but also for them. Acknowledgement and acceptance, however, embrace both the good and the bad we all face and instead of denying its existence, we use its realization to propel us down a path of growth. It allows us to engage with life where it is instead of imprisoning ourselves in victimhood, and wishing for something to be other than it is.

Are you resisting a current toxic reality? Can you begin to look at the situation with curiosity? What pain do you need to acknowledge and accept so you can begin to move forward? Can you let go of the need for your perpetrator to change in order for you to forgive?

2. Compose

Composing a comprehensive, coherent and compassionate narrative that explains your perpetrator's actions and your response is the core of forgiveness. You have already begun the preparation for rewriting your narrative as you clearly elicited and acknowledged the facts and difficult emotions associated with the transgression. A comprehension narrative also includes, however, the inner story of your perpetrator. You can transform your story of victimhood into the story of a victorious hero.

Just before Archbishop Tutu died, Douglas Abrams arranged a multi-day interview with both Tutu and the Dalai Lama. Abrams had the daunting task of distilling the core principles that guided the lives of two of the world's most influential spiritual leaders. His quest was to highlight universal truths that bridged their different worlds of faith. In the end they agreed that joy, and the associated peace that comes with it, is the central, universal desire of all people, and yet it is not something that can be directly achieved. Rather, it is a by-product of living by eight virtues: perspective, humility, humor, acceptance, compassion, gratitude, generosity, and forgiveness. Abrams documented his interview in *The Book of Joy*.

Both men's paths ran through adversity. Tutu's path traversed apartheid's persecution of Black people in South Africa, and the Dalai Lama's path through the Chinese government's attempts to eradicate the culture and faith of the Tibetan people. Adversity and how they learned from it was essential to their understanding of true joy.

Because humans are primarily relational beings, I believe joy is a by-product of our ability to transform our toxic stories into stories of healing. This transformation process is by definition forgiveness, and forgiveness is achieved by infusing the other seven virtues: perspective, humility, humor, acceptance, compassion, gratitude, and generosity into our narratives and our persecutors' narratives. The path looks like this: **Adversity - Infused Virtue - Forgiveness - Joy.**

Let's look at what infusing virtue into adverse relationships looks like.

- **Perspective:** Perspective implies you view the world and time in a way that transcends your self-limited interests. I like to think of this as viewing my life through the eyes of God. You may simply think of it as viewing your life through the eyes of an entity much larger than yourself. I like to walk outside in the early morning hours when it is still dark and I can see the night sky filled with millions of stars. I call this "starry night therapy." It helps remind me that I and all my troubles are minuscule in the grand scheme of things. It broadens my sense of time, importance and complexity.

As I apply this broader sense of perspective to forgiveness, it reminds me that we all see the world differently, and that difference can be helpful. The picture that comes to my mind is that we are all satellites orbiting the earth in fixed positions. Based on our unique life experiences, gifts and genetics, we each see the world only from these different fixed positions. One person may see part of Antarctica, Africa, South America, and the southern Atlantic Ocean.

Another person may see India, Australia, China, part of Russia, and the Indian Ocean. Yet another may see the world as the vast watery Pacific Ocean with a few islands scattered throughout. Who is right? Who sees the world correctly? We are each looking at the same world, but what we see is very different. As limited creatures, we don't have the capacity to see all truth directly, but we can understand truth more broadly when we first seek to understand through the eyes of others. In this way, if we stay curious enough we can stitch together truth as a more complete 360-degree mosaic.

Perspective also reminds me that each of our minds acts as a mosaic. We like to think of ourselves as solitary agents, but as you have discovered, our minds really work like a collective of internal characters. These different inner characters often want diametrically opposed things simultaneously. Part of me may love you and simultaneously part of me may be angry with you. Viewing not only ourselves but others as a mosaic, including those who hurt you, can foster healing and understanding.

Perspective broadens our understanding of time and importance as well. Can you include the totality of your experiences into view as you attempt to explain your life? Can you identify good that has come from your bad experiences? That doesn't mean you should adopt a Pollyanna view of life and ignore the pain you have experienced. It simply means that you can look beyond the pain and include a broader set of experiences. The Dalai Lama explains that without his persecution by the Chinese government, and his subsequent escape and exile, he would never have left the walls of his Potala Palace and been exposed to a much broader world and ways of thinking. As a result, his life has become much richer and more nuanced because of the persecution.

How can you see the world through the eyes of others? Through the eyes of your persecutors? Without negating the hurt you have experienced, what gems of wisdom have you gained or can you begin to see as the result of your trials?

- **Humility:** Connected to the concept of perspective is humility—the ability to fully appreciate others. In South Africa, Tutu explains that the term "ubuntu" means that all people are interconnected and that we receive our humanity through our relationships with others. As I begin to understand you, I begin to understand myself. Separateness leaves us feeling anxious and lonely, but humility fosters a sense of unity and completeness.

Acknowledging that we all not only feel pain, but inflict pain and have the potential for both constructive and destructive emotions broadens our self-centric view of importance. Each of us wants to feel worthy and valued. Each of us wants to be free from suffering. Each of us wants to be filled with peace and joy, and each of us wants to be healthy and happy. We all are striving for these same goals the best we know how with the tools we have at our disposal, but our efforts are imperfect and often leave others hurt in the process.

Understanding and acknowledging that suffering is not unique to us and is part of our shared common humanity is both liberating and uniting. We all can discover a commonality in our struggles. Humility provides us with a healthier perspective of our place in what is and what will be.

Humility also recognizes that our success is not simply the result of our own efforts. I am able to write this book in part because of the nourishment of the food on my table, food that countless people grew, packaged, shipped, and sold. In my small medical practice I don't do everything. Without my wife, who serves as my office manager, and my phlebotomist, "my" practice would never survive.

Humility also recognizes that all our blessings and gifts are from something bigger than ourselves and that eventually all of us will be the one in need.

How can humility change your view of the people who have harmed you? What do you have in common with them? As you think about those who have hurt you, can you remember times when you hurt others? What did it feel like when they forgave you? Can you imagine granting your perpetrator that same feeling?

- **Humor:** I find that I am drawn to people who are able to laugh at themselves, their mistakes and their inadequacies. They don't take themselves too seriously. We all know people who think they are better than everyone else, arrogantly strutting around with their nose in the air. Arrogance ironically arises out of a sense of insecurity and the need to falsely elevate ourselves above others in order to feel better about ourselves. People who are able to laugh at themselves, on the other hand, are secure in their identity, recognizing both their gifts and their limitations.

How can you find humor in your inadequacies? In your ability to relate to others? In your attempts to justify your righteous anger?

How can you use levity to acknowledge your failures as well as soften and de-escalate tension between you and someone you care about?

- **Compassion:** Thupten Jinpa PhD created the Compassion Cultivation Training program at Stanford University and is the author of *A Fearless Heart: How the Courage to be Compassionate Can Transform Our Lives*. Jinpa defines compassion as, "a sense of concern that arises when we are confronted with another's suffering and feel motivated to see that suffering relieved."[103]

Instilling compassion is essential for forgiveness and begins with the process of self-compassion we discussed in Chapter 3. When we don't show ourselves self-compassion and instead base our self-worth on our achievements and the need to defeat others, we discover that there is never a limit to the time and energy we must devote to that never-ending, all-consuming endeavor. As a result, self-care, rest, exercise, and time for meaningful relationships become afterthoughts, subjugated to the need to win. In the end it leaves people feeling anxious, depressed and angry.

According to social scientist Kristen Renwick Monroe, the key component of compassion for others is the ability to perceive all humankind as connected. She refers to this as a, "perception of a shared humanity."[104] Studies show that the ability to see others like ourselves, even in simple ways, fosters a sense of empathy and compassion. The opposite is also true. Inability or unwillingness to perceive similarity has huge implications, and we can see the consequences of ignoring this in the atrocities of the 20th century.

Jinpa explains, "From slavery to the Jewish Holocaust, and from the ethnic cleansing in the Balkans, to the Rwandan genocide, at the root of all these horrors is the lack of perception of a shared humanity. Rather, the victims were subjected to stages of progressive dehumanization, beginning with differentiation of 'us' and

---

103 Thupten Jinpa, *A Fearless Heart: How the Courage to be Compassionate Can Transform Our Lives* (Avery, May 5, 2015).

104 Kristen Renwick Monroe, *The Heart of Altruism: Perceptions of a Common Humanity* (Princeton University Press, 1996)

'them,' objectification, and generalization of the other through stereotyping, dehumanization, and in some cases, demonization."[105]

Recognizing our similarities is often the opposite of what we see in our current national discourse. We segment ourselves into us vs. them, black vs. white, rich vs. poor, gay vs. straight, male vs. female. We stereotype all white males as angry and racist or all gay Black females as beligerant and militant.

We've dehumanized each other, and many are now openly justifying violence as an appropriate way to counter those with whom they disagree. We physically attack each other during protests, scream down dissenting views, vandalize churches, synagogues, homes and businesses, loot innocent peoples' property, and storm the capital all in the name of reparation and justice. I could be talking about Nazi Germany, but I'm referring to the US now.

Civilizations don't begin with the intention of mass genocidal cleansings. It begins with a simple intolerant perspective, refusing to see others as similar to ourselves. More radical views become progressively more palatable as we slowly slide into the quagmire.

The solution is compassion. It begins with how we view ourselves, our family and then extends to our friends, our community, and finally to the wider world. Failure to soothe yourself with compassion or allow yourself to feel your own pain safely creates a heart that can't feel the pain of others. With no way to feel others' pain it becomes easy to justify doing whatever it takes to meet your own selfish needs at others' expense. Dehumanize others and you become the demon we all fear.

Why do we resist compassion if it is so good?

---

105 Thupten Jinpa, *A Fearless Heart: How the Courage to be Compassionate Can Transform Our Lives* (Avery, May 5, 2015)

1. We have adopted a scarcity mindset. We believe we are competing against everyone for everything.

2. We fear experiencing the suffering and pain that can come with emotional vulnerability.

3. We fear receiving compassion from others because we worry they will want something in return.

4. We fear becoming or appearing weak.

While we all have the potential to forgive, it takes time and effort to cultivate. It is much easier to simply blame somebody else.

One way to cultivate those seeds is by repeating a Compassionate Forgiveness Mediation. Like the compassionate meditation I introduced in Chapter 3 which encourages acknowledgement, validation, common humanity, soothing touch, and comforting words, focusing on a meditation that seeks the specific relief of your perpetrator's suffering will help rewire your brain to grow and nurture a heart of forgiveness.

Consider repeating something like this as a prayer or meditation:

- May (the name of your perpetrator) feel worthy and valued.

- May (the name of your perpetrator) be free from suffering.

- May (the name of your perpetrator) be filled with peace and joy.

- May (the name of your perpetrator) be healthy and happy.

If that meditation feels easy, but you are still hesitant to act out your compassion, consider this more active compassionate meditation:

- Assume a calm body position.

- Close your eyes and take a few deep breaths.

- Address any difficult feelings or thoughts you may have.

- Once you feel ready to progress, while you are still taking in slow deep breaths, visualize yourself breathing in your perpetrator's pain and suffering and breathing out compassion for them.

View this as an active prayer or a wish that frees them from suffering. While it can be used as prayer for divine help, it also helps change your attitude toward your perpetrator. By combining the physical movement of your breath with the meditation or prayer, you prime yourself to act out compassion as you directly encounter those who offend and hurt you.

What prayer or meditation can you think of that will nurture forgiveness by encouraging a compassionate heart?

- **Gratitude:** In most situations, strained relationships are the fault of both parties. That is not to say there aren't exceptions, as in the case of rape, murder or other severe abuse. In most normal relationships, however, where loved ones or friends argue, fault is bilateral. Infusing gratitude into the story, especially into your perpetrator's story, can help you recognize and reframe your cognitive distortions, freeing you to see the truth more clearly and to forgive. Consider going back to Chapter 4, reviewing the common cognitive distortions and identifying those that apply to your situation.

One of our most prominent cognitive distortions is our innate negativity bias. From an evolutionary perspective, it makes sense that we are wired this way. It helps us stay cautious and on guard, always looking for predators that can harm us. In modern life, however, always looking through such a narrow lens focuses our attention on people's failures and negative traits while blinding us to the rest of their humanity. It shifts our focus on what has been done wrong and needs to be fixed instead of more comprehensively seeing what has been done correctly and what is right about our relationships.

As we infuse gratitude into our perpetrator's story, we begin to recognize that while they have negative qualities they also have positive traits, and we begin to see their complexity and our commonness. As we infuse gratitude into our own story we bolster our sense of self-worth and self-compassion, lessening our feeling of victimization, decreasing our self-absorption and opening our hearts to a wider social perspective. Our negative thoughts and feelings, as a result, begin to dampen, allowing us to extract previously unrecognized benefits and to see what is most important.

In Chapter 7, I introduced the outline of my Self-Care Journal. Part of that exercise includes writing about three things for which you are grateful each morning, and at the end of the day writing a few sentences about something you discovered, achieved, are thankful for or are excited about. Both are meant to bolster your sense of gratitude.

One of the benefits of gratitude journaling is that it deliberately changes the words we use, which is important because our words create our reality. Words like "giving," "fortune," "satisfaction," "blessedness," and "thankfulness" create an abundance mindset and a grateful attitude. In contrast, words like "deprivation," "regrets," "lack," "need," and "loss" create a scarcity mindset and an ungrateful attitude.

Infusing gratitude into an unhealthy relationship can be emotionally difficult. It forces us to face the reality of our strong uncomfortable emotions and begin to counter them with more expansive language.

How can you modify these gratitude journaling steps to focus on a strained or toxic relationship and infuse positive words and thoughts into it? Can you think of any positive qualities your perpetrator may have? Maybe you are not ready to express gratitude for that person. That's okay. Can you think of anything positive that has happened as the result of your encounter with that person? Can you think of anything positive that person has ever done? Try to write about any of these.

Maybe you are not ready to express gratitude in any way for your perpetrator and can't see any good that has come from your relationship. Nobody has the right to force you through your forgiveness journey faster than you are ready. If you are trying to make progress, that is all anybody can expect.

If you are not ready to infuse your perpetrator's story with gratitude, consider working toward the desire to feel gratitude in some way for them or your situation. If it doesn't seem possible, can you think of a person who has been able to do this, somebody who can serve as an example for you to follow? What did they do? What can you emulate? Consider praying or meditating for the ability to see your situation through a similar lens.

- **Generosity:** The University of Notre Dame's Science of Generosity Project defines generosity as the virtue of giving good things to others freely and abundantly.

The English word generosity is derived from the Latin word "generosus" which means "of noble birth." Up to and including the 16th century, generosity was used to describe a person as being of noble lineage. In the 17th century, it began to denote a nobility of spirit; whether someone possessed various admirable qualities, not a literal family heritage. It embodied the idea that someone's behavior was consistent with the idealized concept of nobility. It wasn't until the 18th century, however, that generosity began to be used according to our modern definition.

While we think of being generous with our thoughts, words, money, time, things, and attention, I think the concept of the 17th century definition is still pertinent—and the most important. As we freely and abundantly give, we share an even greater gift: a noble spirit. This generosity of spirit, which includes your attitudes and emotions, is contagious.

The human brain is equipped with a specialized type of neuron called mirror neurons which allow us to automatically feel what others are feeling and infer intentions by watching others' behaviors and reactions. As you walk into a room, your mood—positive or negative—is subconsciously transmitted to everyone you encounter. Virtues are indirectly transmitted through this emotional connection. People emulate the ways of behaving and relating they find attractive. One of the greatest gifts you can give, therefore, is an ennobling spirit that lifts up and affirms others through compassion, humility, acceptance, gratitude, and forgiveness.

By nature I am introverted. I have learned to engage people, but mingling in crowds does not come naturally. I can do it, but it is an energy-consuming process. On the flip side, I am energized by thinking in quiet solitude. As a result, I was intensely shy when I was younger. It wasn't until I was a teenager that I met somebody who helped me change.

Tom Young was the music minister in my church. He was a vivacious character with an infectious laugh. People of all ages were drawn to him. In the small town where I grew up, there were not a lot of positive social activities for young people. Our church's youth choir was one of them. It was a popular place to be on Sunday afternoon, in large part because of Tom. He loved kids and freely showed it.

Tom saw potential in me. He recognized a rudimentary singing talent and by nurturing that helped me gain confidence not only in singing, but—more importantly—in my ability to engage with people. With his contagious personality and the emotional power of music he taught me that the heart of a relationship is an emotional connection. While I wasn't extroverted like him, I discovered that I could emotionally connect in meaningful ways and that people were longing for these kinds of connections.

At the time I thought Tom was focusing his attention on me, but in reality he was that way with everybody. He was just being himself and in doing so he made me feel special. I was fortunate to find somebody who believed in me and whose love of life and generosity were so contagious.

Tom gave me a precious gift that I still savor today, some forty years later. The practice of generosity is, however, not only about what you give others. It also is about what you get in return, or should I say, what you become in the process. Generosity is an ennobling path that helps you grow into a person concerned with things bigger than yourself.

In social media, it seems people focus on rights, retribution and reparation. People want to know, "What will I get?" instead of, "What can I give?" Unfortunately, in these types of discussions people become so blinded by anger, distrust and envy that they miss a great truth: generosity is ennobling, and selfishness is embittering.

Do you need to infuse the story of someone who has harmed you with generosity? Not for their sake, but for who you became in the process. Has your current inability to forgive left you embittered? What do you need to give generously in order to free yourself from these chains?

3. Forge

Forge a new type of relationship by either renewing it in a new healthier way or releasing it.

Webster's Dictionary defines *forgiveness* as, "To cease to feel resentment against an offender; to give up resentment of or claim to requital (something given in return, compensation or retaliation.)"[106]

Acknowledging, accepting and composing a new narrative that explains your conflict and your perpetrator's inner story is the path to this traditional definition of forgiveness and to healing the inner turmoil in your heart. It is the path to releasing the need for your perpetrator to change, for the past to be different from it was and for your need for retaliation or seeing your perpetrator harmed. As stated before, forgiveness does not mean that you do not seek justice. It does not mean that you don't try to stop your perpetrator. It does not mean that you condone the wrongdoing, and it does not mean that you forget the offense. But what happens once you have done all that? What do you do with the remnant of the relationship? This is what most people don't discuss, especially when they gloss over forgiveness with the simple "forgive and forget" mantra.

The path to forgiveness extends beyond the traditional definition of forgiveness. It goes beyond simply changing your heart. Forging recognizes that the relationship is disrupted, that it has been injured and is in need of being rebuilt in some way. But how do we go about rebuilding the relationship in a newer, healthier way that will help prevent the same thing from happening again and that honors each person's common humanity?

What this new version of your relationship looks like depends on four factors:

- How successful you were in the first phases. Have you been able to give up your need for retaliation and the need for the past to be different than it was? How emotionally resilient have you be-

---

106 "forgiveness" Merriam-Webster.com. 2022. https://www.merriam-webster.com (1 September 2022).

come? Have you worked through the steps of awareness, attenuation, assets, allies, and aim, and begun to take action on these? The degree to which you can lead yourself effectively with perspective, humility, humor, acceptance, compassion, gratitude, generosity, and forgiveness will determine how safe you will be if the relationship once again turns toxic.

- The second is the degree to which your perpetrator takes responsibility for their actions, acknowledges the facts and emotional harm they have caused and seeks to make restitution to the degree that is possible.

- The third factor includes the severity and chronicity of the offense. If your offender said something like, "You're a jerk!" one time and has otherwise been loving and considerate, you shouldn't find it too difficult to renew that relationship completely and quickly. Moving along the spectrum, you may have been in a relationship where your perpetrator emotionally abused you for years, but never physically harmed you. Renewing that relationship is possible and preferred, but will take a lot more work on both your parts. On the other end of the spectrum, your perpetrator may have murdered a loved one, is not sorry for doing it and has threatened to kill you if they get a chance. The relationship you forge with that individual is obviously different from the relationship you forge with the person who hurt your feelings.

- The fourth factor is the type of relationship you have with your perpetrator. Are they a family member, a friend, an acquaintance or a stranger? If you decide to release the relationship with a close family member like a parent, a spouse or sibling, there are more consequences than releasing a relationship with a stranger.

In a perfect world, both you and your perpetrator would successfully work through your own forgiveness paths and rebuild a new relationship that better honors healthy boundaries. Tutu calls this renewing the relationship. Renewing is always the ideal and preferred way of reassembling the pieces of a broken relationship. It is built on mutual respect and a commitment to the wellbeing of both parties.

On the opposite end of the spectrum, if you are in the early stages of developing resiliency or your perpetrator shows no remorse, you may need to release yourself from the relationship. If your perpetrator is a close family member or friend, hopefully you distance yourself from the relationship only long enough for you to become more resilient and for them to take responsibility for their actions. Permanently releasing the relationship may be the healthiest option, however, when a stranger has acted in an intensely malicious way and has no intention of taking responsibility.

Forging is a continuum that runs between **renewing** and **releasing**, with complete renewal on one end and permanent release on the other. In reality, most conflicts don't lie on the extremes and most often involve people we care about. In these situations, forging is a process that takes time. Forging a new relationship might involve releasing yourself from the relationship for a period while you calm your emotions, build resilience and learn to lead yourself in healthier ways. If you remember from Dr. John Gottman's Love Lab, it takes people about thirty-sixty minutes to calm their body's response to conflict and begin to think more clearly and rationally. In minor conflicts, you may only need to release the relationship for a few minutes while you compose yourself. With chronic and more intense conflicts, you may need a lot more time, maybe weeks or months, to sort through your feelings and thoughts. As with the other stages of forgiveness, that's okay. Take the time you need to work through your difficult emotions, and don't let anybody rush you. With close relationships, the preferred goal is to eventually renew the relationship.

It is important to note that this renewed relationship does not mean you return to the same old, abusive relationship. It means you lead yourself with confidence, courage and clarity and that you protect and provide for yourself while requiring respect for newer, healthier boundaries. It also means that you acknowledge your own role in the conflict, how you may have inflicted pain and how you need to make restitution to the degree possible.

Healthy relationships are never final destinations; they remain works in process. The moment you stop growing and changing is the moment the relationship stagnates. One word of caution: if you release yourself from a toxic relationship with a close relative or friend, try not to permanently give up on the relationship. If part of your justification for distancing yourself is that you don't trust your loved one to act respectfully or appropriately, ask yourself whether you also don't trust yourself to adequately protect and provide for yourself, enforce healthy boundaries and speak the truth when it becomes uncomfortable. If so, challenge yourself to grow and become such a better version of you that despite your loved one's best efforts, or lack of effort, you become strong enough to unilaterally renew the relationship. If you fail, at least you will have grown and will rest well knowing that you did everything possible to appropriately repair the relationship.

The Dalai Lama says, "You can accept that your relationship with your neighbor is difficult and that you would like to improve it. You may or may not succeed, but all you can do is try. You cannot control your neighbor, but you do have some control over your thoughts and feelings. This is the only chance to improve the relationship. In time, maybe they will become less difficult. Maybe not. This you can not control, but you will have your peace of mind."[107]

---

107 Dalai Lama, Desmond Tutu, and Douglas Carton Abrams, *The Book of Joy: Lasting Happiness in a Changing World* (Avery, September 20, 2016).

Only you can decide whether it is most appropriate to renew or release the relationship.

Updated Concept of Growth

In Chapter 5, I introduced the concept of growth as a function of the intensity of adversity and the strength of your skill set. (Figure 8.1)

When the two are closely matched, we grow. When they are disproportionate, we either feel overwhelmed or stagnate. Whether we actually take action to change and overcome our challenges is a little more complicated.

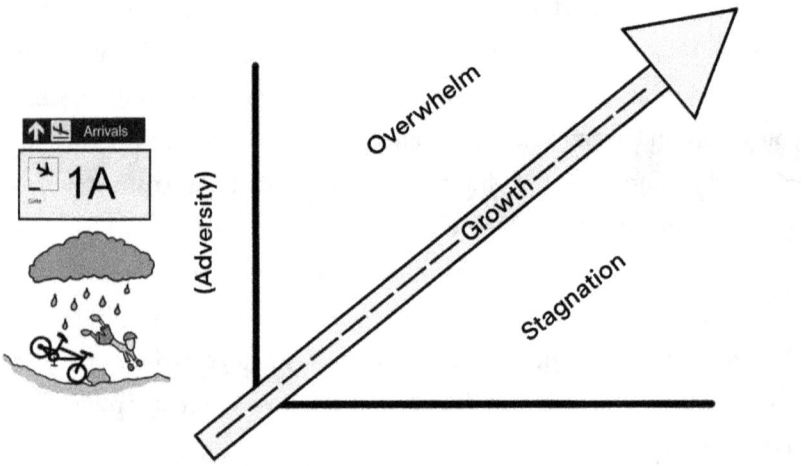

(FIGURE 8.1)

Cast your mind back to the Motivational Interviewing process we learned about in Chapter 6. This is a powerful clinical approach that helps people unlock their internal resources for change. Drs. Miller and Rollnick, who developed this clinical approach, believe people are born with an innate drive to flourish, and that change is a function of our strengths and how important the proposed change is to us. They go on to explain that importance is a factor of how well the proposed change correlates with your most important values. Degree of motivation, therefore, is determined by our strengths and values.

As Archbishop Tutu and the Dalai Lama suggest, positive values—or virtues—are not something the majority of us spontaneously manifest. Instead, they must be instilled through practical application. As we discussed earlier in the chapter, this is an effortful process that occurs as we infuse these virtues into our stories.

How do we decide on which values to base our motivation system, since not all values promote positive change? After reviewing the science of change and thousands of years of sacred teachings, I believe compassion is the central virtue that grounds all others in a healthy motivation system. Compassion helps us discover a healthy middle ground or balance between providing for our own needs while also providing for others' needs. Tutu and the Dalai Lama made the argument that compassion, perspective, humility, humor, acceptance, gratitude, forgiveness, and generosity are universal virtues of joy. You can make the argument that these virtues can serve as an excellent starting point. You can also make the argument to include others like love, joy, peace, patience, kindness, goodness, faithfulness, gentleness, and self-control or compassion, calmness, curiosity, connection, courage, confidence, clarity, and creativity. Whichever list you choose, use compassion as the core virtue that links all the others. For me, Archbishop Tutu's and the Dalai Lama's list makes sense.

I like to visualize this process as wrapping myself with a cloak of ennobling virtues, which fits the theme of our inner victorious hero.

As we leap into action and don the ennobling cloak, our outer character changes and our deep inner characters transform. Our beliefs and attitudes expand and grow, freeing us to do the difficult work of caring for ourselves and others.

This updated concept of growth looks like this:

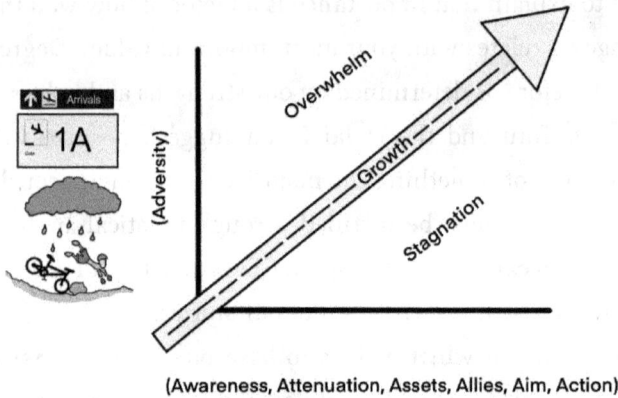

(Awareness, Attenuation, Assets, Allies, Aim, Action)

+

1. Perspective   5. Compassion
2. Humility   6. Gratitude
3. Humor   7. Forgiveness
4. Acceptance 8. Generosity

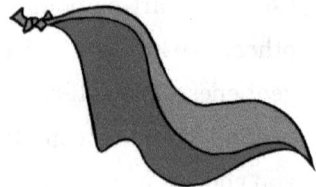

(FIGURE 8.2)

Transformation from victim to a victorious hero is an intentional, active process which mirrors how our brain encodes memories into different levels of understanding.

1. Verbal understanding (explicit or declarative knowledge.) Simple facts.

2. Critical understanding. Through deep reflection, meditation or visualization, simple facts become integrated into our overall fund of knowledge.

3. Embodied understanding (procedural or implicit knowledge.) Through repetitive application, verbal understanding or explicit knowledge integrates into our automatic Deep Brain's pathways and alters the way we respond, believe and emote.

With simple concepts like riding a bicycle, you may skip the middle step, but it starts by understanding the basics of how a bicycle functions. This head knowledge or verbal understanding, however, does not automatically translate into embodied knowledge, so the first time you tried to ride your bike you probably crashed. It wasn't until you applied your verbal understanding repeatedly that it integrated into your Deep Brain and you finally rode your bike successfully.

More complex concepts integrate the middle step as well. While learning to fly an airplane is similar in many ways to learning to ride a bicycle, it is obviously much more complex. I began studying aviation years before I began my flying lessons. I learned avian physics, weather patterns, principles of combustion engines, how electrical systems work, radio communication techniques, and more. My brain was full of facts, and I aced the written exam. The first few weeks of practical training, however, were ugly. My Surface Brain was completely overwhelmed with all the things I had to simultaneously do.

I was trying to consciously control the plane's speed, direction and elevation; monitor critical engine parameters; monitor the plane's progress over the ground; look for emergency landing spots; and communicate with the tower through a new garbled abbreviated language. I was mentally exhausted after my first few flights. With repetition, I integrated all the pieces and my Deep Brain began to take over some of the tasks, freeing my Surface Brain to focus its attention only on the most critical ones.

When I transitioned to instrument training, which is even more rigorous, we added another step, the flight simulator. In the flight simulator I visualized and practiced some of the basic physical procedures like pushing/pulling throttle knobs and steering with the yoke while only referencing the airplane's flight gauges. It provided a safe environment for me to practice as my Deep Brain learned these new repetitive procedures. Meditation and visualization for Empowered Self-Care work in a similar manner. While simulator work and meditative/visualization practices are helpful, neither is exactly the same as the real thing. Explicit knowledge fully integrates into our Deep Brains only when we apply it repeatedly in the real world.

This process is bidirectional. Our thoughts and understandings shape how we perform or act, and our actions also shape the way we think, store and use information. This is extremely helpful. Sometimes life can be so confusing we don't know what to do. We feel paralyzed. One solution is to simply take action. Do something positive. Do something constructive. As you take action, your Deep Brain encodes that action into embodied understanding (procedural knowledge) which in turn guides your future ways of thinking and acting.

Sometimes when I have a patient who feels overwhelmed, we begin the empowerment process by simply picking pleasant behaviors for them to do a few times a week. From a list of 365 pleasant activities, I ask them to choose one or two that resonate with them or to use the list to foster their own creative ideas. The activities are simple like daily walking, meeting a friend for lunch, lying in the sun or arranging flowers. With these simple activated behaviors, people begin to think and feel more positive which boosts their confidence and empowers their sense of inner strength.

As Terry and I visit, he acknowledges that Empowered Self-Care has already broadened his understanding of himself in many critical ways, and yet he is concerned that this path of forgiveness is more than he can manage. I remind him that forgiveness is a path we may never fully conquer, but we can choose to walk daily. It is a path of small, consistent steps, and as with all journeys it progressively builds on our successes. These small, active steps not only progress tangible successes, but they also rewire our deep neurologic thinking patterns which shape our future thoughts and behaviors.

"If we're facing in the right direction,
all we have to do is to keep on walking."[108]

"Don't bend the truth or say things that you know
are not right. Keep your eyes on the path and look
straight ahead. Make sure you are going the right way,
and nothing will make you fall."[109]

The Dalai Lama's and Archbishop Tutu's stories remind us that infusing virtues into our difficult stories is not always an easy task. Hurt people often react unkindly. It takes courage to lower your defenses and to reach out to hurt people where they are and show them love, compassion and forgiveness.

Terry notices that as he begins to infuse virtue into his difficult narratives, his attitude softens and he begins to remember happier

---

108 Joseph Goldstein, *The Experience of Insight: A Simple and Direct Guide to Buddhist Meditation* (Shambhala; Reissue edition. October 24, 2017).

109 Proverbs 4:24-26.

stories from his childhood. Good memories tend to fade in the presence of anger and resentment. Dr. John Gottman discovered this in his Love Lab. When relationships turn toxic, couples' shared positive storylines fade. He also noticed that this process is often reversible as couples forgive and re-establish fondness and compassion for each other. Terry is experiencing this as happier memories from his childhood begin percolating to the surface.

Terry's confidence is steadily increasing. He understands that external adversities don't automatically equate to internal suffering and that he can depart from his self-induced toxic ways of reacting if he stays focused on the right path. He reminds himself that he is much stronger than when we first began his journey. Picturing forgiveness as a process of infusing ennobling virtues into his difficult stories helps foster motivation because it links the importance of doing so to a set of positive values that make sense to him. He acknowledges that it is a journey he will be on for the rest of his life. He decides to embrace his discomfort and embark on this new part of the journey.

As he continues to cloak himself, and the stories of his parents, with compassion, acceptance and generosity, he begins to recognize a commonality with their struggles. He begins to see them more broadly as people who had not only induced pain, but also as people who were suffering and didn't know how to alleviate their own pain. Terry also sees himself more broadly in the relationship as someone who has both experienced and caused pain. Humility reminds him that he is no better than them, and that without the tools of Empowered Self-Care he has been trapped in a toxic recirculating prison. He is grateful that he has been shown the way, and acknowledges that his parents never had that advantage. Terry shares that he thinks part of his journey is now to reveal this path to them, not through words, at least not initially, but by the way he lives and how he reinterprets his image of them and others. He begins to understand that we all are on our own versions of this path, and hopefully as we become better versions of ourselves, we emerge from our own trials better equipped to provide for ourselves and others.

Terry would tell you that his journey is still a work in progress, but this final step of infusing virtues into his difficult stories is the piece that helps release himself from his destructive thoughts and emotions. It allows him to face the other stages of Empowered Self-Care with more curiosity, clarity and confidence.

In this final phase of Action, as he puts all the components into place, he begins to understand the broader implication of Empowered Self-Care. When we keep our eyes on the path and intentionally take action to walk the right way, we experience healing for ourselves. In the process, we also become a better version of ourselves that helps heal our family, friends and community. In this way, we all are connected and dependent on each other. This path releases us from our old stories of victimhood and transforms them into victory.

The Final Question

Mortimer Adler's challenge to us in the Preface is now your question to answer:

If you find this author's message compelling and true, then you must ask, "What will I do about it?" or "What now?"

Knowing information without acting is of little value. As Adler said, "Nothing short of the doing solves the problem."[110] Psychologists often say that you can't think yourself to health; you must do something.

Your ticket to a better, more beautiful life is free ...

---

110 Mortimer Adler and Charles Van Doren, *How to Read a Book: The Classic Guide to Intelligent Reading* (Touchstone, 1940).

Boarding Pass — Empowered Self-Care — Boarding Pass

First Class

Username: _____

Destination: Beautiful Life   Current Location: Reality

Arrival: **Gate 1A** (Adversity)

Departure: **Gate 6A** (Awareness, Attenuation, Assets, Allies, Aim, Action)

← ✈ Departures

✈ **6A**
Gate

Boarding Pass — Empowered Self-Care — Boarding Pass

Sword of Truth
1. Alternatives
2. Evidence
3. Implications
4. Observation
5. Usefulness

Cloak of Virtue
1. Perspective
2. Humility
3. Humor
4. Acceptance
5. Compassion
6. Gratitude
7. Generosity
8. Forgiveness

www.DrYou.org

✈ **6A**
Gate

The question is, will you redeem it?

DR. YOU

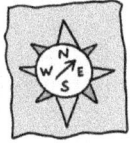

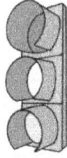

(Awareness)

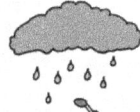

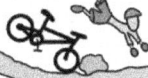

(Adversity)

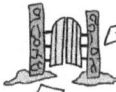

(Attenuation)

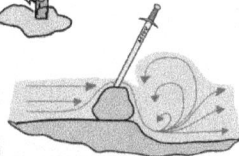

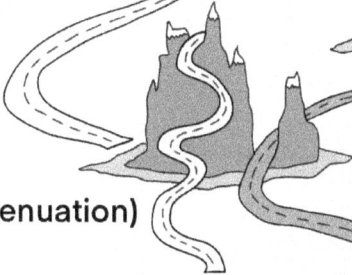

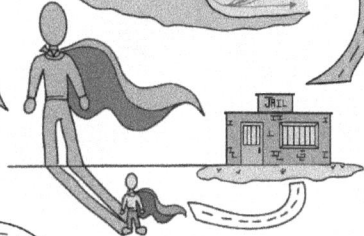

(Assets)

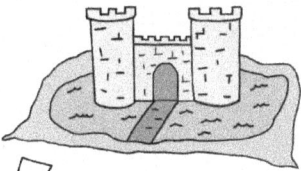

(Allies)

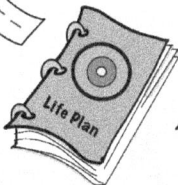

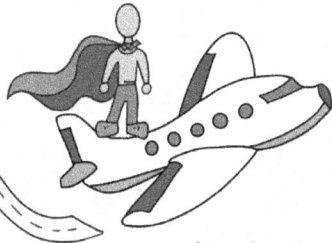

(Aim)

(Action)

Hope to see you on the path!

APPENDIX I

Recommended Reading

1. *Man's Search For Meaning* - Viktor Frankl

2. *The Hero With a Thousand Faces* - Joseph Campbell

3. *Maps of Meaning* - Jordan Peterson

4. *The Coddling of the American Mind: How Good Intentions and Bad Ideas Are Setting Up a Generation for Failure* - Greg Lukianoff and Jonathan Haidt

5. *Thinking, Fast and Slow* - Daniel Kahneman

6. *Dopamine Nation: Finding Balance in the Age of Indulgence* - Anna Lembke

7. *Feeling Great: The Revolutionary New Treatment for Depression and Anxiety* - David B. Burns

8. *Willpower: Why Self-Control Is the Secret to Success* - Roy F. Baumeister and John Tierney

9. *Worldwide Laws of Life: 200 Eternal Spiritual Principles* - John Marks Templeton

10. *The Happiness Hypothesis: Putting Ancient Wisdom to the Test of Modern Science* - Jonathan Haidt

11. *Internal Family Systems Therapy* - Richard Schwartz

12. *Competing Against Luck: The Story of Innovation and Customer Choice* - Clayton M. Christensen

13. *The Person Called You: Why You're Here, Why You Matter & What You Should Do With Your Life* - Bill Hendricks

14. *The Marshmallow Test: Understanding Self-Control and How to Master It* - Walter Mischel

15. *The Worry Cure: Stop Worrying and Start Living* - Robert L. Leahy

16. *Cognitive Behavioral Therapy Made Simple: 10 Strategies for Managing Anxiety, Depression, Anger, Panic, and Worry* - Seth J. Gillihan

17. *The Body Keeps The Score: Mind, Brain and Body in the Transformation of Trauma* - Bessel van der Kolk

18. *The Hope Circuit: A Psychologist's Journey from Helplessness to Optimism* - Martin E. P. Seligman

19. *Bandersnatch: C. S. Lewis, J. R. R. Tolkien, and the Creative Collaboration of the Inklings* - Diana Pavlac Glyer

20. *The Storied Nature of Human Life: The Life and Work of Theodore R. Sarbin* - Karl E. Scheibe and Frank J. Barrett

21. *Churchill: Walking With Destiny* - Andrew Roberts

22. *The Last Lion: Winston Spencer Churchill: Visions of Glory, 1874-1932* - William Mancester

23. *A Dancer in Wartime: One Girl's Journey from the Blitz to Sadler's Wells* - Gillian Lynne

24. *The Element: How Finding Your Passion Changes Everything* - Ken Robbins et al

25. *How to Have a Good Day* - Caroline Webb

26. *Positivity: Groundbreaking Research to Release Your Inner Optimist and Thrive* - Barbara Fredrickson

27. *12 Rules for Life: An Antidote to Chaos* - Jordan Peterson

28. *The Social Brain: Discovering the Networks of the Mind* - Michael S. Gazzaniga

29. *The Seven Principles for Making Marriage Work* - John M. Gottman

30. *Stanley: The Impossible Life of Africa's Greatest Explorer* - Tim Jeal

31. *The One Thing: The Surprisingly Simple Truth Behind Extraordinary Results* - Gary Keller

32. *Story: Substance, Structure, Style and the Principles of Screenwriting* - Robert McKee

33. *Positive Psychotherapy* - Tayyab Rashid and Martin P. Seligman

34. *Quality of Life Therapy: Applying a Life Satisfaction Approach to Positive Psychology and Cognitive Therapy* - Michael B. Frisch

35. *How to Read a Book: The Classic Guide to Intelligent Reading* - Mortimer J. Adler and Charles Van Doren

36. *The Artist's Way: A Course in Discovering and Recovering Your Creative Self* - Julia Cameron

37. *The Book of Joy: Lasting Happiness in a Changing World* - Dalai Lama and Desmond Tutu

38. *The Book of Forgiving: The Fourfold Path for Healing Ourselves and Our World* - Archbishop Desmond Tutu and Rev. Mpho Tutu

39. *A Fearless Heart: How the Courage to Be Compassionate Can Transform Our Lives* - Thupten Jinpa

40. *The Master and His Emissary: The Divided Brain and the Making of the Western World* - Iain McGilchrist

41. *The Matter With Things: Our Brains, Our Delusions, and the Unmaking of the World* - Ian McGilchrist

42. *All My Road Before Me: The Diary of C. S. Lewis, 1922-1927* - C. S. Lewis

Pleasant Activities

- Soaking in the bathtub

- Planning my career

- Getting out of (i.e. paying on) debt

- Collecting things

- Going on vacation

- Thinking how it will be when I finish school

- Taking deep breaths

- Recycling old items

- Going on a date

- Relaxing

- Going to a movie in the middle of the week

- Jogging or walking

- Thinking I have done a full day's work

- Listening to music

- Buying household gadgets

- Lying in the sun

- Laughing

- Thinking about my past trips

- Listening to others

- Reading magazines or newspapers

- Hobbies

- Spending an evening with good friends

- Planning a day's activities

- Meeting new people

- Remembering beautiful scenery

- Saving money

- Going home from work

- Eating

- Practicing karate, judo or yoga

- Thinking about retirement

- Repairing things around the house

- Working on my car or bicycle

- Remembering the words and deeds of loving people

- Wearing sexy clothes

- Having quiet evenings

- Taking care of my plants

- Buying or selling stock

- Going swimming

- Doodling

- Exercising

- Collecting old things

- Going to a party

- Thinking about buying things

- Playing golf
- Playing soccer
- Flying kites
- Having discussions with friends
- Having family get-togethers
- Riding a motorcycle
- Sex
- Running
- Going camping
- Singing around the house
- Arranging flowers
- Practicing religion
- Losing weight
- Going to the beach
- Thinking I'm an okay person
- A day with nothing to do
- Going to reunions
- Going skating
- Going boating
- Traveling abroad or in the US
- Painting
- Doing something spontaneous
- Doing needlepoint, knitting or cross-stitch
- Sleeping
- Driving

- Entertaining
- Going to clubs
- Thinking about getting married
- Going hunting
- Singing with groups
- Flirting
- Playing musical instruments
- Doing arts and crafts
- Making a gift for someone
- Buying records
- Watching boxing or wrestling
- Planning parties
- Cooking
- Going hiking
- Writing short stories, novels, poems or articles
- Sewing
- Buying clothes
- Going out to dinner
- Working
- Discussing books
- Sightseeing
- Gardening
- Going to the beauty parlor
- Early morning coffee and newspaper
- Playing tennis

- Kissing
- Watching children play
- Thinking I have a lot more going for me than most people
- Going to plays and concerts
- Daydreaming
- Planning to go to school
- Thinking about sex
- Driving or taking a train cross-country
- Listening to the stereo
- Refinishing furniture
- Watching TV
- Making lists of tasks
- Going bike riding
- Walks in the woods or at the waterfront
- Giving gifts
- Traveling to national parks
- Completing a task
- Watching football, hockey or baseball
- Eating a favorite food
- Teaching
- Photography
- Going fishing
- Thinking about pleasant events
- Playing with animals
- Flying a plane

- Reading fiction

- Acting

- Spending time by yourself

- Writing diary entries or letters

- Cleaning

- Reading nonfiction

- Taking children places

- Dancing

- Going on a picnic

- Thinking "I did that pretty well" after doing something

- Meditating

- Playing volleyball

- Having lunch with a friend

- Going to the mountains

- Thinking about people I like

- Thoughts about happy moments in my childhood

- Splurging

- Playing cards

- Solving riddles

- Having a political discussion

- Playing softball

- Seeing or showing photos or slides

- Playing guitar

- Doing crossword puzzles

- Shooting pool

- Dressing up and looking nice
- Reflecting on how I've improved
- Buying things for myself
- Talking on the phone
- Going to museums
- Thinking religious thoughts
- Lighting candles
- Listening to the radio
- Getting a massage
- Saying "I love you"
- Thinking about my good qualities
- Buying books
- Taking a sauna or a steam bath
- Going skiing
- Whitewater canoeing or rafting
- Going bowling
- Doing woodworking or carpentry
- Fantasizing about the future
- Taking ballet or tap dancing classes
- Debating
- Sitting in a sidewalk café
- Having an aquarium
- Going horseback riding
- Thinking about becoming active in the community
- Doing something new

- Making jigsaw puzzles
- Thinking I'm a person who can cope
- Being in the country
- Making contributions to religious, charitable or other groups
- Talking about sports
- Meeting someone new
- Listening to live music
- Planning trips or vacations
- Rock climbing or mountaineering
- Reading the scriptures or other sacred works
- Going to service, civic or social club meetings
- Rearranging or redecorating my room or house
- Being naked
- Reading a "How to Do It" article or book
- Reading stories, novels, poems or plays
- Going to lectures or hearing speakers
- Writing a song or a piece of music
- Saying something clearly
- Doing something nice for my parents
- Restoring antiques
- Talking to myself
- Working in politics
- Working on machines
- Completing a difficult task
- Solving a problem, puzzle or crossword

- Laughing
- Going to a celebration
- Shaving
- Having lunch with friends or associates
- Taking a shower
- Riding in an airplane
- Exploring the wilderness
- Having a frank and open conversation
- Thinking about myself or my life
- Speaking or learning a foreign language
- Going to a business meeting or a convention
- Being in a sporty or expensive car
- Cooking
- Being helped
- Wearing informal clothes
- Combing or brushing my hair
- Taking a nap
- Canning, freezing and making preserves
- Solving a personal problem
- Being in a city
- Singing to myself
- Making food or crafts to sell or give away
- Playing chess or checkers
- Doing craftwork (pottery, jewelry, leather, beads or weaving)
- Scratching myself

- Putting on makeup

- Designing or drafting

- Visiting people who are sick, shut in or in trouble

- Cheering or rooting for someone

- Being popular at a gathering

- Watching wild animals

- Having an original idea

- Landscaping or yardwork

- Reading professional literature

- Wearing new clothes

- Just sitting and thinking

- Seeing good things happen to my family and friends

- Going to a fair, carnival, circus, zoo or amusement park

- Talking about philosophy

- Planning or organizing something

- Listening to the sounds of nature

- Dating or courting

- Having a lively talk

- Having friends come to visit

- Playing sports

- Introducing people who I think would like each other

- Getting letters, cards or notes

- Watching the clouds, sky or a storm

- Going on outings to the park, a picnic or a barbecue

- Giving a speech or a lecture

- Reading maps
- Gathering natural objects (rocks or driftwood)
- Working on my finances
- Wearing clean clothes
- Making a major purchase or investment
- Helping someone
- Getting promoted
- Hearing jokes
- Talking about my children or grandchildren
- Going to a crusade
- Talking about good health
- Seeing beautiful scenery
- Eating good healthy meals
- Improving my health (having my teeth fixed, getting new glasses, changing my diet)
- Doing a job well
- Having spare time
- Loaning something
- Being noticed as sexually attractive
- Making others happy
- Counseling someone
- Going to a health club
- Learning to do something new
- Thinking about my parents
- Supporting causes I believe in

- Kicking leaves, sand or pebbles

- Playing lawn sports (badminton, croquet, bocce, horseshoes)

- Seeing famous people

- Going to the movies or renting a film

- Budgeting my time

- Being praised by people I admire

- Feeling a spiritual presence in my life

- Doing a project in my own way

- Doing odd jobs around the house

- Crying

- Being told I am needed

- Being at a family reunion or get-together

- Giving a party

- Washing my hair

- Coaching someone

- Going to a restaurant

- Seeing or smelling a flower or a plant

- Being invited out

- Receiving honors

- Using perfume, cologne or aftershave

- Having someone agree with me

- Reminiscing about old times

- Getting up early in the morning

- Having peace and quiet

- Doing experiments and other scientific work

- Visiting friends
- Playing football
- Being counseled
- Saying prayers
- Giving a massage
- Taking adult education courses
- Doing favors for people
- Talking with people I enjoy
- Being asked for help or advice
- Helping other people solve their problems
- Playing board games
- Sleeping soundly at night
- Snowmobile or dune buggy riding
- Being in a support group
- Dreaming at night
- Playing ping-pong
- Brushing my teeth
- Walking barefoot
- Playing frisbee or catch
- Doing housework or laundry
- Petting and necking
- Amusing people
- Going to a barber or hair stylist
- Having houseguests
- Being with someone I love

- Sleeping late
- Starting a new project
- Being assertive
- Going to the library
- Playing rugby or lacrosse
- Birdwatching
- Shopping
- Playing video games or going to an arcade
- People watching
- Building or watching a fire
- Selling or trading something
- Finishing a project or task
- Apologizing
- Learning a new computer skill
- Being a leader
- Being with happy people
- Playing games
- Writing cards or notes
- Asking for help or advice
- Talking about my hobbies or special interests
- Smiling at people
- Playing in sand, a stream or the grass
- Expressing my love to someone
- Talking with friends over coffee or tea
- Playing handball, paddleball or squash

- Surfing the internet

- Remembering a departed friend or loved one, visiting the cemetery

- Staying up late

- Going skiing or snowboarding

- Having family members or friends do something that makes me proud of them

- Going to auctions or garage sales

- Thinking about an interesting question

- Doing volunteer work or working on community service projects

- Water skiing, surfing and scuba diving

- Defending or protecting someone; stopping fraud or abuse

- Hearing a good sermon

- Winning a competition

- Making a new friend

- Reading cartoons, comic strips or comic books

- Borrowing something

- Traveling in a group

- Seeing old friends

- Mentoring someone

- Using my strength

- Attending an opera or the ballet

- Playing with pets

- Looking at the stars or the moon

- Being coached

About The Author

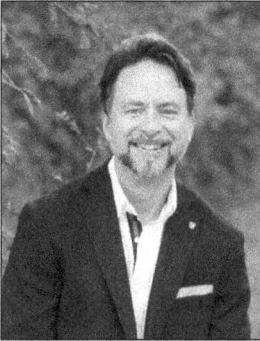

Dr. David Ball is an internal medicine physician, author, and podcaster. He holds a Bachelor of Science in Biology from Baylor University, a Medical Doctorate from the University of Mississippi, and completed his Internship and Internal Medicine Residency at the University of Tennessee in Chattanooga. Dr. Ball established and runs a relationship-centric outpatient medical practice, Dr. David Ball Concierge Care (www.drdavidball.com), a boutique physical training center, Life Changing Fitness (www.LCFTyler.com), and an online health and wellness community / resource center, Fit For Impact (www.fitforimpact.com), as part of a more comprehensive and hemispherically balanced approach to health. He is an outdoor enthusiast who enjoys mountain biking, road cycling, hiking, backpacking, and traveling. He lives with his wife and children in Tyler, Texas.

For questions and requests for speaking engagements contact info@drdavidball.com.

www.ingramcontent.com/pod-product-compliance
Lightning Source LLC
Chambersburg PA
CBHW071234290326
41931CB00038B/2961